Vitamins & Minerals for a Healthy Pregnancy

This book is dedicated with much love to my wife, Robbie, and our very healthy son, Michael.

Vitamins and Minerals for a Healthy Pregnancy

How the right foods and nutrients can help you and your baby

Richard Gerson Phd

Foreword by
Douglas Hall MD

Arlington Books
King Street, St. James's
London SW1

VITAMINS AND MINERALS FOR
A HEALTHY PREGNANCY
*First published in the United States of America
this edition published 1987 by
Arlington Books (Publishers) Ltd
15-17 King Street, St. James's
London SW1*

Copyright © 1987 Richard Gerson

*Typeset by Rapidset & Design Ltd., London
Printed and bound by
Biddles Ltd., Guildford*

British Library Cataloguing in Publication Data

Gerson, Richard
Vitamins and minerals for a healthy pregnancy.
1. Pregnancy—Nutitional aspects
2. Vitamins in human nutrition
I. Title
613'.04244   RG559

ISBN 0–85140–715–3

Contents

Foreword, 7
Douglas Hall MD

Introduction, 9

1 Nutrition for a Healthy Pregnancy, 13

2 Vitamins and Minerals, 22

3 Exercise and Pregnancy, 76

4 Summary, 88

5 Questions and Answers, 89

Publisher's Note

The guidelines in this book are not a substitute for professional medical care during pregnancy. The information provided should be applied in consultation with your doctor.

Foreword

It has been my experience that the half dozen things that make a difference in the quality of your pregnancy are the major components of wellness. *What is wellness?* Wellness is an alternative to doctors, medicines, hospitals and disease. Wellness in pregnancy is the state of expectant mothers who are operating at or near their potential because of the lifestyle they have adopted *before and during* their pregnancies. Your present state of well-being reflects the many lifestyle decisions you have made up to this point in your life. The components of wellness are: *nutritional awareness, physical fitness, stress management, self-responsibility, environmental sensitivity, and spirit.*

Your baby's life is just beginning as it grows within you. *Your* lifestyle decisions will affect the health of your baby! You wouldn't expect a perfect seed to grow into its greatest potential in less than ideal soil, and your baby is no different. The true potential of the miracle growing within you may not be realized if you don't understand the principle of the seed and the soil.

Keeping the above factors in mind what steps are necessary to assure that the requirements of the seed and the soil are fulfilled, so that you may enjoy your pregnancy and a beautiful, healthy baby?

Think of yourself as an artist. You are the one painting the picture. Each moment of your life is a moment of creation for yourself and your baby. It is impossible to develop every opportunity, so now you must focus on the opportunities that will be potentially beneficial to you and your developing baby. *Knowledge* is the key. You may not be able to do all that you learn, but at least learn all that is possible. How sad it would be to come to the end of your pregnancy, and then discover something that you could have done to make it a more rewarding experience for you and your baby. You may not like all that you learn, but that's life. Your baby has to rely on your learning and applying the appropriate knowledge anyway.

What are the total requirements of the seed and the soil? You don't want to spend a lot of time on minor things! Concentrating on minor details keeps many expectant mothers from having a less than ideal pregnancy. I recall one expectant mother who was concerned about taking aspirin, while ignoring the fact that she smoked a pack of cigarettes a day!

My experience tells me that expectant mothers learn because of one of two reasons, inspiration or desperation. This foreword, and the book that follows, is not only meant to serve as a source of inspiration, but as a source of knowledge that you may use for your benefit.

This book presents a difficult subject so that you learn what is important to prepare your body, so that your baby will have the nutrients that are needed for optimal development. This is important information that you can readily understand. The requirements for each nutrient, its function in your body and your baby's body, the potential effects of excess or deficiencies, and the natural source of the nutrient are presented in a concise manner. The quality of your baby's life may depend on the knowledge you gain from reading this book.

Douglas C. Hall MD

Introduction

Pregnancy is one of the most natural and beautiful occurrences in a woman's life. For many it is more than just the creation of a new life. It is the fulfillment of a dream, an expression of true love, and the culmination of the natural instinct to be a parent. But pregnancy is not always an easy road. There are abundant physiological and psychological changes that a woman undergoes both during and after pregnancy. It is imperative that all future mothers be prepared for these changes.

Everything a woman does affects her unborn child. These effects are set in motion even before she becomes pregnant. What she thinks, what she feels, what she does, and, most importantly, what she eats all influence the development of the unborn child. This point cannot be overemphasized. *Everything a mother does affects her baby!*

This book will focus on the relationship between vitamins and minerals and a healthy pregnancy. That does not mean that a mother should be concerned about supplementation or basic nutrition only after she becomes pregnant. She should be concerned about her nutritional status before she becomes pregnant. It is a well-documented fact that a mother's prepregnant nutritional state has a great influence on the growth and development of the baby. Additionally, the mother's nutritional state and eating habits during pregnancy will also have a dramatic effect on the child. After all, the only nutrition the baby receives is through the mother, and we all know that output is a function of input. If you eat well and do the things you should do during pregnancy, you will probably have a healthy baby. If you don't feed yourself properly, the foetus will start to feed from your food stores and reserves. This will weaken you and then both you and your baby may suffer from nutritional deficiencies.

This book is designed to prevent that from happening. It is a guide to a healthy pregnancy through the proper intake of vitamins and minerals. It is important to remember that vitamins and minerals are not food replacements; they are food supplements. Their function is to make the mother's metabolism more effective, so that the foods she eats are transferred to the baby efficiently.

The book also contains information on basic nutrition, good eating habits during pregnancy, and special nutritional needs during pregnancy. This is not a nutrition text, nor is it meant to be a comprehensive analysis of all the factors related to pregnancy. The book is intended to serve as a reference source for pregnant mothers who are interested in improving the level of their nutrition so that they may do the same for their unborn baby.

The main section describes the many vitamins and minerals that may have a positive influence on pregnancy. There is a description of each vitamin and mineral, including where it comes from, the beneficial effects it has in relation to pregnancy, what can happen during pregnancy if you are deficient in it, and what some of the best food sources are for that vitamin or mineral. There are also summary charts that show the Recommended Dietary Allowance (RDA) for each vitamin and mineral, its best food sources, deficiency symptoms related to pregnancy, and how the vitamin or mineral can best benefit pregnancy during a given 3 month period.

A short final section describes how exercise relates to pregnancy. Recent research has shown that exercise during pregnancy, under proper supervision and adhering to appropriate standards and guidelines, can have a beneficial effect on the mother without harming the foetus. In fact, as the mother's circulatory and respiratory systems improve with exercise, the transfer of nutrients to the baby will also improve. Furthermore, exercise during pregnancy enables a mother to withstand the strain of labour and delivery better and return to her prepregnant shape and physical fitness more quickly.

This book, in general, explains the benefits of a wellness-oriented lifestyle for pregnant women. This lifestyle should be maintained before, during, and after pregnancy to ensure a healthy baby and a healthy mother. There is additional information on how best to determine your supplementation needs, plus some suggestions about vitamins and minerals for the newborn. Finally, charts in the appendix provide quick reference for everything discussed in the book.

Remember that this is a guidebook. *It is not a substitute for professional medical care during pregnancy. The information provided is based on the latest research and scientific facts, but only you and your doctor know how the material described here best applies to you.* Vitamin and mineral supplements in the proper dosages can have a highly beneficial effect on you and your baby. That is the goal of this book: to provide enough information so that you can become a wise consumer and take vitamins and minerals properly to help you and your baby.

1

Nutrition for a Healthy Pregnancy

Proper nutrition is the most important factor in a healthy pregnancy. It is more important than childbirth education classes, exercise, or almost anything else. Good nutritional habits can overcome almost any previous bad habits, such as alcohol or smoking. Perhaps the only thing that good nutrition can't overcome is critical illness, yet there is more and more research today that points to the remarkable effects of positive dietary practices on apparently "terminal" conditions.

Only good nutritional practices can maintain your health and assure that your baby will have an adequate birthweight and normal growth and neuromuscular development. Childbirth education classes teach pregnant women and fathers-to-be what to expect during pregnancy and how to handle labour and delivery. This is important to ease the stresses and uncertainties associated with pregnancy. Exercise is also important because it helps you stay in shape and provides you with the strength necessary for a successful labour and delivery. However, nutrition, more than these two factors or anything else, determines how well you will feel and react during pregnancy. It is also your nutritional habits that will determine how healthy your baby will be at birth.

If you are in good health, exercise, and have an adequate reserve of all the necessary nutrients before you become pregnant, you will experience a pregnancy with fewer complications than a woman who is undernourished or malnourished when she becomes pregnant. That does not mean that a women whose pre-pregnant nutritional habits were poor will not be able to remedy the situation. On the contrary, the body responds rapidly to positive changes in nutrition, and so does the baby.

There are several important nutritional factors that will affect the outcome of a pregnancy. These include your pre-pregnant nutritional status, your nutritional habits during pregnancy; the severity of a nutritional deficiency, should it occur, and its duration; and the stage of gestation during which the deficiency occurs. These factors were suggested almost twenty years ago by the U.S. Committee on Maternal Nutrition (1970), and they are still valid today. We know from research with animals and from observing human births that poor nutrition results in smaller babies; babies with lower birthweights; premature births; reduced head circumference (which may mean reduced brain development); physical and mental handicaps that may not be obvious at birth but that may appear later in life; more complications during pregnancy, labour, and delivery; and 'in some severe cases' maternal and foetal death. There is even speculation that poor nutrition may be a cause of Sudden Infant Death Syndrome (cot death) because of poor development of foetal organs.

The most common consequence of improper nutrition is a low-birth weight baby. This is easily overcome by a diet that is adequate both in caloric quantity and nutritional quality. A proper diet will allow you to gain between 24 and 30 pounds during pregnancy, with the baby weighing in at about 7 pounds at birth. The 24 to 30 pounds is just a range to consider. If you are a thin person, you may be able to gain more weight during pregnancy. Conversely, if you are overweight, you don't have to gain so much weight. Ideally, overweight women should lose some weight and get closer to their recommended body weight before becoming pregnant. However, no pregnant woman should ever go on a reducing diet. Restriction of calories also means a restriction in nutrients. This leads to a reduction in the quantity and quality of nourishment that the foetus receives. The mother who eats properly during pregnancy should experience the following breakdown of weight gain:

	lbs
Breasts	0.5 (each)
Body Fluids	2.5
Increased Blood Volume	4.0
Body Stores	3.5
Total Weight Gain	approx. 24.0

Obviously, the only way to achieve this weight gain is to eat more than you normally would. You are truly eating for two. It is recommended that you consume approximately 300 calories a day more than you normally would. If you regularly eat 1,500 calories a day, you should eat at least 1,800 calories a day while you are pregnant. The extra energy that comes from the additional calories helps you sustain yourself during the day and also nourishes the foetus.

There is another reason that calories intake must increase during pregnancy. Your requirements for specific nutrients, as well as the baby's need for similar nutrients, increases as the pregnancy continues into the last 3 months. More and more energy is needed to move the larger body mass and nourish the growing foetus. Thus, the wise mother-to-be will develop a food plan that not only calls for an increase of about 300 calories a day but also makes certain that she and her unborn baby are receiving the proper nutrients.

Nutrients

Nutrients are divided into two categories: macronutrients and micronutrients. The micronutrients comprise carbohydrates, proteins, and fats. The micronutrients are vitamins and minerals. A third, and separate category of nutrient, is water.

Carbohydrates

Carbohydrates are the primary energy source of the body. They provide approximately two-thirds of an individual's total energy needs. Carbohydrates come in two forms: simple and complex. We know these as sugars and starches. Usually, carbohydrate foods that are high in sugar, such as biscuits, cakes, and pies, are relatively low in nutritional value for the calories they contain. On the other hand, starchy or complex carbohydrate foods such as vegetables, bread, and potatoes contain a great many nutrients in their calories. Complex carbohydrates are also a good source of dietary fibre, or roughage, Fibre goes through the digestive system essentially intact and helps the body eliminate waste products and function smoothly. Whole grains, fruits, and beans, in addition to the other complex carbohydrate foods already mentioned, are excellent sources of fibre.

Carbohydrates provide the body with its initial source of energy for any activity. They are broken down and stored in the muscles and liver as glycogen. They are released into the system as soon as "instant energy" is required. The problem is that we do not eat enough carbohydrates. While consumption of fruits and vegetables has increased in the last few years, we still do not get enough of our calories from them. Part of the problem is that fatty foods taste so good. The other and perhaps more important part is that carbohydrates have received bad publicity.

We were told that foods such as pasta, potatoes, and breads were not good to eat because they led to weight gain. That is one of the greatest fallacies in nutrition. Actually, a diet high in complex carbohydrates is best suited for any type of weight-control programme, whether it is gain, loss, or maintenance. A diet high in simple carbohydrates *will* lead to weight gain because of the empty calories, which are calories that have little nutritional value. You should make certain, therefore, that your diet consists of adequate amounts of complex carbohydrates to ensure that you have enough energy throughout pregnancy, labour, and delivery.

Protein

Proteins have been called the building blocks of life. Proteins are essential to the function and maintenance of every cell in the body. That includes the daily activity of your body as well as that of the growing foetus. Proteins also serve as regulators of chemical reactions that keep the body growing and working properly. For example, protein is used to formulate red blood cells, new body tissues, muscles, bones, and even the milk for breast-feeding. The importance of protein in a pregnant woman's diet cannot be overemphasized. That is not to suggest that women overcompensate in their protein intake. Many people already eat more protein than they really need. Rather, it is important that you consume the right amounts of protein for yourself and your baby.

In America the Food and Nutrition Board of The National Academy of Sciences recommends a daily protein intake of between 70 and 80 grams for pregnant women. However, there are nutritional professionals who consider this amount too low and suggest that you consume 90 to 100 grams of protein every day, especially during the last half of the pregnancy. Only you and your doctor can determine the exact amount of protein that is right for you based on your body size, prepregnant weight, rate of weight gain, and the size of your baby. Protein deficiency can harm both you and your baby. It can lead to an underproduction of brain cells in the foetus, the development of weak bones and teeth, and an overall slowing of the child's growth patterns. A mother whose diet was deficient in protein can compensate during her pregnancy by eating adequate amounts of protein every day.

Proteins are made up of and broken down into amino acids. These are the true building blocks of life. Scientists have identified more than twenty amino acids. The body produces all but eight of these. These eight are called essential amino acids and must be supplied by food. Complete proteins, such as those found in meat, fish, eggs, and dairy products, contain all eight of these amino acids. Incomplete proteins, such as those in vegetables and vegetables products, lack one or more of the essential amino acids. However, two or more incomplete proteins, or an incomplete and a complete protein can be combined to provide all the required amino acids.

There is one important point to remember about protein consumption. Many of the best sources of protein are also high in fat. In fact, it is not uncommon for most of the calories in a high-protein food to come from the fat in that food. So, when you choose the protein foods for your pregnancy diet, choose carefully and wisely.

Fats

High-fat foods are a boon to the fast-food industry and a bane to the eating public. Currently, in the 'civilised' West we consume almost 40 percent of our calories from fatty foods. That is extremely unhealthy because we know that fat can lead to many terminal diseases. We must understand that the body can manufacture much of the fat it needs from the carbohydrates and proteins we consume. Whenever we eat an excess of calories, regardless of the type of food it is, the body stores the excess fat. Therefore, it is wise, even during pregnancy, to reduce fat consumption to about 30 percent of total calories. This is healthier for you and your baby because more nutrients are then supplied by carbohydrates and proteins.

These negative aspects are not meant to imply that fat is unimportant in the body. Fat is required for many vital functions. Fat supports and cushions organs, provides insulation against extreme heat or cold, becomes the primary energy source when exercise continues for long periods of time, provides the oils in the body that keep the skin and hair moist, and aids in the production of prostaglandins, the fatty acids that help regulate the body's use of cholesterol. Without fat, your hormone balance and menstrual cycle would be disrupted. Finally, fat is required for the absorption and utilization of certain vitamins, specifically A, D, E, and K. These roles for fat are the same whether you are pregnant or not. It may be that some of these functions, such as protection and vitamin utilization, become more important during pregnancy.

Vitamins and Minerals

Vitamins are organic compounds that have no caloric or energy value. They serve as catalysts in all the complex nutritional chemical reactions that occur in the body. These reactions known collectively as metabolism, are responsible for converting fats and carbohydrates into energy, helping protein build new and repair injured tissue, and allowing the body to function to meet the demands of daily living. There are both fat-soluble and water-soluble vitamins, and each has a specific function that will be discussed in detail in the next section.

Minerals are chemical substances that participate in many of the chemical reactions that are essential to human nutrition and proper body functioning. Minerals do not provide energy, but they do act as components of major body structures, including bones, teeth, and soft tissues. Some of the more important minerals in pregnancy are iron, calcium, potassium, and sodium. While it is possible that a prepregnant woman may not need vitamin and mineral supplements, most pregnant women require supplements to the nutrients they receive from their diets.

Water

Water is perhaps the most vital of all nutrients. The entire body is a fluid medium, and all the cells require water to function. Water makes up 60 to 70 percent of our bodies. In addition to being the primary component of all cells, including blood, water is involved in the transport of nutrients throughout the body. Water is also responsible for regulating body temperature, especially under conditions of extreme heat or cold.

It is vitally important for you to consume six to eight eight-ounce glasses of water each day. This benefits both you and your baby. Water in your system helps you to produce blood continuously, which carries nutrients to the placenta and into the fetus. Furthermore, the natural stress of being pregnant may induce body temperature changes, and water helps maintain a normal body temperature. Adequate water consumption is even more important if you exercise during your term. Since exercise depletes body fluids, it is imperative that you replenish the fluids by drinking enough water to quench your thirst and then drinking some more. Remember, just because you quench your thirst does not mean you have satisfied your cells' need for fluid, or your baby's needs.

Food Groups

Most of us are familiar with the Basic 4 food groups. They are milk and dairy products, meat products, vegetables and fruits, and breads and cereals. Some authorities have suggested further dividing these groupings into five, seven, and in some instances, nine food groups. While this may facilitate clinical diet counselling, it can become confusing. Therefore, for our purposes, we will consider the standard Basic 4. The chart in Appendix A shows these food groups and how many servings from each you should eat daily. These suggestions are merely guidelines, and your actual consumption may vary depending on the type of pregnancy, your health status, and the recommendations of your doctor. The important thing is to be sure that you get enough of the proper foods from each group to provide you with a balanced diet.

Summary

This chapter has provided an overview of nutrition and how it relates specifically to pregnant women. Many people follow the Recommended Dietary Allowances (RDAs) to determine the nutritional adequacy of their food intake. However, some nutritionists and professional dieticians recommend even higher intakes of all nutrients than the levels specified by the

RDAs. There are figures in Appendix A that show the recommendations of both. The best way to determine your personal needs is to meet with your doctor, develop a sound food-management programme that can be followed throughout your pregnancy, and take supplements as directed. This will usually ensure a safe and healthy pregnancy for you and your baby.

2

Vitamins and Minerals

The importance of vitamin and mineral intake during pregnancy cannot be overemphasized. There is considerable research, both in animals and humans, that describes the destructive effects of malnutrition or nutrient deprivation on the birthweight and overall development of the foetus. We know that nutritional deficits in the mother lead to developmental deficits in the baby. Thus, our primary concern should be how to guarantee that you receive an adequate amount of all the vitamins and minerals that you and your baby need.

Some of the required amounts of nutrients can come from a well-balanced diet, while others, such as iron and folacin, must come from supplements. It is not our purpose to become involved in the long-standing controversy over whether or not sufficient amounts of vitamins and minerals come from a well-balanced diet, or whether cooking and processing wash away these nutrients, making supplements necessary. Instead, this chapter will describe all the vitamins and minerals that are necessary for a healthy pregnancy.

A Primer on Vitamins

Vitamins are organic compounds found only in living things or the products of living things. All known vitamins are found in varying quantities in specific foods. Each vitamin is essential for proper health, growth, and development.

Unfortunately, the body is not capable of synthesizing all vitamins; most must be provided through dietary means or supplementation.

Vitamins work with protein to assist in the digestion of food, the provision of nutrients to all cells in the body, and the production of energy. Vitamins initiate chemical reactions that allow other hormones and enzymes to complete their work. It is easy to see why a deficiency of one or more vitamins can lead to certain symptoms.

The amount of vitamins a woman should consume has been established through the Recommended Dietary Allowances (RDA). The RDAs are the amounts of vitamins that prevent deficiency diseases. However, there is considerable controversy as to whether the RDAs are sufficient to promote health, as opposed to merely warding off disease. The resolution of the controversy is beyond the scope of this book. It may not be relevant, though, because nutritional requirements increase during pregnancy to levels that usually exceed the RDAs. Some women will need more of a particular vitamin during pregnancy than others, so every pregnant woman must establish her own "RDA" with the help of her doctor.

It is certain that all the vitamin needs of a pregnant woman cannot be met through food consumption alone. Vitamin supplements are necessary to offset any possible deficiency. However, proper supplementation is the key, because megadoses can produce the same type of harmful effects as deficiencies.

Vitamins are classified as either fat-soluble or water-soluble. The fat-soluble vitamins are A, D, E, and K, with some authorities classifying fatty acids as vitamin F. The water-soluble vitamins are the B complex and C. Fat-soluble vitamins can be stored in the body, while water-soluble vitamins cannot. Therefore, it is especially important during pregnancy to consider the type of vitamin, when to take it, and how much to take. The type of vitamin and how much you should take can be determined by your doctor.

The best time to take vitamins is after a meal. This enables better absorption and helps the body to utilize each vitamin better. Additionally, the fat-soluble vitamins can be stored in the fat from the food. Most well-balanced diets are not rich enough in all the vitamins and minerals, and you need and should consider proper supplementation under the guidance of your doctor.

Vitamin A

Benefits to Your Baby: Aids bone and tissue growth and cell development. Maintains health of skin and mucous membranes for mother and baby throughout pregnancy.

Vitamin A is a fat-soluble nutrient that occurs either as preformed vitamin A in the tissues of animals or as carotene, which must be converted into vitamin A before it can be used by the body. Carotene is abundant in carrots, hence its name. Folklore tells us that if we eat carrots we will be able to see better at night. This is more truth than folklore. Carrots are an excellent source of vitamin A, which is known to prevent night blindness. While the prevention of night blindness is the most well-known benefit of vitamin A, it is only one of the many important functions performed by that vitamin.

Vitamin A is instrumental in the growth and repair of body tissues and it helps maintain smooth, soft, disease-free skin. Vitamin A helps protect the mucous membranes that line the mouth, throat, nose, and lungs. This reduces the body's susceptibility to infection. Hence, vitamin A is important to the functioning of the immune system. The vitamin also helps protect the digestive tract, kidneys, bladder, and other visceral organs. Finally, vitamin A is involved in the building of strong bones and teeth, the formation of red blood cells, the development of good eyesight (both day and night), and the production of RNA, which is the nucleic acid that transmits instruments within all cells on how they must function for optimal health.

Vitamin A is also important for foetal development during pregnancy. All the benefits mentioned above apply to both you and your baby. Your serum levels of vitamin A decrease in early pregnancy, rise during late pregnancy, fall during labour, and rise again after delivery. These fluctuations are also affected by foetal need and storage of the vitamin. That is why the RDA of vitamin A for pregnant women is 5,000 IU (International Units), which is a 25 percent increase over the requirements for nonpregnant women.

During pregnancy, vitamin A easily passes through the placenta to the foetus. Thus, if you are getting enough vitamin A, so is your baby. The vitamin is normally available in adequate supply from the foods you eat, but sometimes supplementation is necessary. This will occur when certain factors, such as excessive alcohol consumption or the use of some drugs, interfere with the body's ability to absorb vitamin A. The vitamin is primarily absorbed in the intestines and stored in the liver. The importance of the relationship between vitamins and minerals is readily seen with vitamin A because an adequate supply of zinc must always be available for the liver to mobilize the vitamin. Another factor that determines the body's ability to use vitamin A is stress. Each person reacts to stress differently, and one of these reactions may involve an inability to utilize vitamin A properly. Pregnancy is a stressful condition because of the demands it places on your body, so it will affect how you absorb and use vitamin A. The RDA of 5,000 IU may have to be adjusted for each individual.

An insufficient supply of vitamin A results in several deficiency symptoms. Some of these may affect your pregnancy and others will just affect you without harming the foetus. Some of these symptoms are vision problems, dry eyes, sties on the eyelids, prematurely aged skin (rough and dry), skin blemishes, loss of sense of smell, loss of appetite, frequent fatigue, and diarrhoea. It is also possible for the hair to lose its lustre and sheen, for dandruff to accumulate, and for the fingernails to become brittle. Even more severe symptoms are the softening of bones and teeth and the loss of the body's ability to absorb vitamin C. This last symptom has far-reaching implications in pregnancy because vitamin C helps you absorb adequate amounts of iron, which prevents anaemia both in you and the foetus.

Some of the more tangible benefits of vitamin A include a strong immune system to prevent illness. If an infection has already occurred, therapeutic doses of the vitamin may keep the infection from spreading. Vitamin A is also important in the cellular repair process, controlling dermatitis, relieving bronchial asthma, reducing high cholesterol into female sex hormones, and possibly even in reducing the risk of cancer. Finally, vitamin A has been used externally as a local application in the treatment of acne, impetigo, boils, open ulcers, and wounds. The vitamin speeds up the healing process, and this is because of its interaction with zinc, which has been shown to be the primary mineral involved in healing.

Overdosing or megadosing on vitamin A can be *extremely dangerous* for pregnant women because it can cause renal and central nervous system damage to their unborn child. It is important to realise with all vitamins and minerals, but primarily with the fat-soluble vitamins, that just because some is good, more is not necessarily better. Most women can get all the vitamin A they need from the foods they eat, such as green and yellow fruits and vegetables, milk products, carrots, and fish liver oil, to name some common sources. If you do not eat these foods or your doctor discovers you have an inability to absorb or utilize the vitamin A in foods, then proper supplementation would be recommended. You should consume adequate amounts of the vitamin throughout pregnancy.

Vitamin B Complex

Benefits to Your Baby: Nervous system development and energy metabolism.

Vitamin B complex consists of a variety of water-soluble

vitamins that are found mostly in brewer's yeast, vegetables, and whole grains. These vitamins include B1 (thiamine), B2 (riboflavin), B3 (niacin), B5 (pantothenic acid, or pantothenate), B6 (pyridoxine), B12 (cobalamin), B15 (pangamic acid), biotin, choline, folic acid (or folacin or folate), inositol and para-aminobenzoic acid (PABA). They are grouped together as the B complex because they share many functional relationships and come from similar sources.

The primary function of the B complex vitamins is metabolic. They help the body convert the macronutrients—carbohydrates, proteins and fats—into energy. The most important metabolic process for the B vitamins involves carbohydrates. Another function of the B vitamins is to ensure the development of a healthy nervous system. Finally, the B complex is involved in maintaining the health of the eyes, hair, mouth, liver, and skin.

The B vitamins should be taken together to ensure maximum benefit. They work synergistically; that is, each one helps the others perform. The reason for this is that they are supplied in the foods mentioned previously as a compound. One B vitamin never exists alone. Another point to remember, especially if you are taking supplements, is that the B vitamins should all be taken in similar doses. Too much of one can cause another to function improperly or not at all.

It is readily apparent how important the B vitamins are to your health and to your developing foetus. Both of you require the conversion of foodstuffs into energy; both require a healthy and properly functioning nervous system; and both, but especially the foetus, require healthy skin, hair, eyes, etc. The problem with pregnancy and the vitamin B complex is that the vitamins' water solubility causes them to be excreted regularly. This also happens in nonpregnant women, but pregnant women show a greater decline in their blood levels of the B vitamins than any other group of people. Matters are further complicated because the foetal levels and requirements of vitamin B complex may exceed maternal levels and supply. Therefore, it is imperative that you continually replace your B vitamin supply.

Another reason you should replenish your B vitamins is that the processing of foods in the typical western diet removes most of them. Women who are irritable, tired, nervous, or even depressed may be that way because of a vitamin B complex deficiency. Pregnant women are also advised not to consume alcohol and sugar. These calorically dense, low-nutrition foods require B vitamins from other parts of the body to metabolize them. The mother's level of vitamin B complex drops, and the baby does not get an adequate supply. The negative feelings mentioned above may being to surface, unobservable problems in the development of the foetus may occur, and the harmful cycle to mother and baby will continue. The solution is to be certain that both you and your baby receive adequate amounts of vitamin B complex.

There are more than a dozen vitamins in vitamin B complex. Each will be described individually along with its benefits to pregnancy, its RDA, food sources, and some of the deficiency symptoms that may occur if there is not enough of the vitamin in your system.

Thiamine (B1)

Benefits to Your Baby: Determines the rate at which energy is released from glucose.

Thiamine affects almost every major organ in the body, including the brain, heart, eyes, ears, stomach, and nervous system. The vitamin is a coenzyme that plays a vital role in the energy production process. Thiamine is primarily responsible for glucose metabolism, which, put simply, is the conversion of carbohydrates into energy. Other functions of B1 are the absorption of neurotransmitters (hormones that help the nervous system work properly), an increase in the potential for learning, and an improvement in the muscle tone of the stomach, intestines, and heart. Two other beneficial effects of thiamine are a consistent growth pattern in children and the possible prevention of plaque accumulation on arterial walls.

Thiamine cannot be stored in the body; it must be replenished daily to provide all these benefits. The vitamin is excreted in the urine in amounts proportional to its ingestion. It is also depleted by consumption of sugar, alcohol, and by smoking. This is not to suggest that B1 deficiencies are common; they are rare. If a deficiency does occur, it would manifest itself as beri beri, which is a disease of the peripheral nervous system. Other deficiency symptoms include appetite loss, anaemia, congestive heart failure, constipation, digestive disturbances, diarrhoea, fatigue, irritability, nervousness, nausea, shortness of breath, and an increased susceptibility to stress. A deficiency symptom more closely related to pregnancy is the inability to digest carbohydrates. This will lead to a decrease in mental alertness, possible cardiac damage to either the mother or foetus, and an inability to transfer needed energy across the placenta.

The RDA for pregnant women is about 1.5-1.6 mg. This may not seem like much, but it is usually enough to prevent any deficiency problems. Foods such as brewer's yeast, brown rice, fish, meat, nuts, poultry, wheat-germ, and whole grain cereals are all excellent sources of thiamine. However, since most of the vitamin B complex is lost in the processing and cooking of foods, supplements may be necessary to reach the recommended levels. This is especially true for pregnant women, who tend to excrete urine more often than nonpregnant women.

Riboflavin (B2)

Benefits to Your Baby: Aids in energy and protein metabolism. Aids in the cell's ability to utilize oxygen and in the maintenance of eyes, hair, nails, and skin.

Riboflavin is important because it is heavily involved in the breakdown and utilization of carbohydrates, proteins, and fats. Riboflavin is also the coenzyme that promotes cellular respiration, which is the ability of each cell to utilize oxygen. Some other functions of vitamin B2 include the metabolism of vitamin C and the maintenance of the eyes, hair, nails, and skin. It is readily apparent that both you and your baby will benefit from an adequate supply of riboflavin.

The problem is that the amount of vitamin B2 in foods is so minimal that it is difficult to obtain even the RDA amounts without taking supplements. The RDA for pregnant women is 1.5-1.8 mg, and although the vitamin is found in conjunction with the other B vitamins in the same food sources, it is not found in large amounts. Hence, the need for supplementation.

Some of the riboflavin deficiency symptoms are diabetes, diarrhoea, indigestion, a lack of stamina and vigour, and possibly a retardation of the growth and development process. The diabetes is related to the role of B2 in the metabolism of carbohydrates, and the growth retardation is due to the body's inability to provide cells with oxygen. Both you and your baby will suffer if you have a B2 deficiency. Another common B2 deficiency problem that pregnant women should be aware of is that they may suffer from eye abnormalities, such as vision problems, burning eyes, and watering eyes.

Because riboflavin is instrumental in the metabolic process, it is also involved in weight gain and weight loss. Weight problems for pregnant and nonpregnant women usually result from an excessive intake of calories. These calories usually come from fat. An over indulgence in fatty foods increases the body's need for riboflavin to support the metabolic processes. If there is insufficient vitamin B2, fat is deposited in various organs of the body, including the arteries. Another source of diet-induced riboflavin deficiency is protein insufficiency. This puts additional stress on the system and forces the adrenal glands to work harder and eventually become overworked. The result is an increased susceptibility to stress and a decreased ability to produce red blood cells. These are the last things a pregnant woman needs. Both of these negative consequences will be detrimental to the developing foetus.

The simplest answer is to eat a well-balanced diet that includes nuts, molasses, brewer's yeast, and organ meats, and to supplement that diet with all the B vitamins. Remember that B complex supplements must contain similar doses of each of the individual vitamins. While this may help you and your unborn baby during pregnancy, you must also be careful after the baby is born. Many babies suffer from jaundice, for which the treatment is phototherapy. Phototherapy involves the use of light, and light tends to destroy riboflavin in the body. So you must make sure your baby gets enough riboflavin. This may be possible through food alone, especially if the infant is breast-feeding. If not, some form of supplementation will be required.

Niacin (B3)

Benefits to Your Baby: Involved in energy and protein metabolism. Effective in improving circulation, removing cholesterol from the circulatory system, and insuring proper function of the nervous system.

Niacin is one of the most important B vitamins for achieving optimum health. Niacin serves many functions, including acting as a coenzyme in the metabolism of carbohydrates, proteins and fats, and aiding in cellular respiration. Niacin is also effective in improving circulation, removing cholesterol from the circulatory system, ensuring the proper function of the nervous system, and aiding in the formation of healthy skin. Niacin also has a positive effect on the development and function of the brain and liver.

Small amounts of niacin are found in many foods, such as lean meats, poultry, fish, liver, wheat-germ, and peanuts.

Thus, we would expect to take in adequate amounts of niacin by eating a well-balanced diet. Unfortunately, that is not always the case; niacin deficiencies can occur. The primary manifestation of deficiency is pellagra, which is characterized by the three Ds: dermatitis, diarrhoea, and dementia. Other signs of this deficiency include depression, fatigue, high blood pressure, nervous disorders, and skin eruptions. Taking too much niacin can result in a "niacin flush," in which skin temperature increases, the face reddens, and blood pressure temporarily drops. Dizziness may also occur.

Niacin has many beneficial effects for pregnant women and their foetuses. The primary functions of the vitamin—metabolism, cellular respiration, nervous system and brain development—all attest to the importance of niacin to a healthy pregnancy. You should take in 15-20 mg of niacin daily. This will provide you with an adequate supply and also allow your baby to receive whatever niacin it needs.

Niacin can be produced by the body from the amino acid tryptophan. Niacin also comes in another form, niacinamide. Niacin itself comes from plants, while niacinamide is found in animals. The human body rapidly converts niacin to niacinamide, which is identical to niacin in every respect except that it does not produce the niacin flush. If you are concerned about receiving adequate supplies of niacin from your food, use niacinamide as a supplement to avoid any possible harmful effects.

Pantothenic Acid (B5)

Benefits to Your Baby: Helps handle stress. Assists in production of adrenaline.

Pantothenic acid is one of the B vitamins that is widely distributed in all living cells. It can be found in yeasts, organ meats, brewer's yeast, egg yolks, and whole grain cereals. Its importance is monumental, as it is the vital part of coenzyme A required for metabolism. Every cell in the body depends on pantothenic acid for its functioning. This is especially true of the adrenal cortex, which produces adrenaline. This hormone determines how well the adrenal cortex responds to stress. The entire body must be mobilized for action, and foods must be quickly metabolized for energy. Pantothenic acid is necessary for these reactions.

A deficiency of pantothenic acid results in the body being unable to respond effectively to stress. The system can no longer utilize vitamin C properly. Vitamin C levels are dependent on pantothenic acid levels. When these levels are low, vitamin C is depleted. If a stressful situation occurs, vitamin C may almost totally disappear from the body.

The liver and the entire immune system are activated when the body is under stress. Pantothenic acid determines how well they respond. There are several other potential disorders that may occur if pantothenic acid is deficient. These include growth problems, depressed antibody formation, spinal cord deterioration, and adrenal insufficiency, to mention a few.

The importance of pantothenic acid to a healthy pregnancy is readily apparent. Both you and your baby must be able to withstand the stress associated with the entire course of pregnancy, labour, and delivery. Also, the development of the internal systems of the foetus are heavily dependent on the amount of pantothenic acid it receives. The recommended daily dosage for pregnant women is 5-10 mg, but there have been suggestions that increased doses are beneficial. You should not exceed 50 mg a day, even though there is no specific range for toxicity of this vitamin.

Pyridoxine (B6)

Benefits to Your Baby: Helps control nausea. Essential for foetal growth. Acts as a coenzyme in amino acid metabolism and protein synthesis. May prevent heart disease.

Pyridoxine is one of the most versatile vitamins in the B complex. This vitamin aids in the absorption of B12, the production of the hydrochloric acid used in digestion, the breakdown of food into usable nutrients, the production of antibodies and red blood cells, and the release of glycogen from the liver for energy. Vitamin B6 may also act as a preventative agent in heart disease. Other functions of pyridoxine include the conversion of the amino acid tryptophan into niacin, the regulation of body fluids by maintenance of the system's sodium-potassium balance, and the synthesis of DNA and RNA. These functions are vitally important to everyone's health, but there are several functions of pyridoxine that are especially significant for women.

Pyridoxine is capable of alleviating problems that include menstrual irregularity, premenstrual tension, skin disorders, pill-induced depressions, and certain complications of pregnancy. The vitamin has also been known to prevent birth defects, aid in the treatment of childhood mental illness, and cure convulsive disorders that may occur during infancy. The importance of B6 to pregnant women is apparent based on its role with DNA and RNA, its coenzyme effect in metabolism, its preventative effect with heart disease, pregnancy complications, and birth disorders, and its role in cellular activity, specifically with amino acid and energy production.

A deficiency of pyridoxine can lead to many problems. Some of the more severe include improper development and functioning of the nervous system in infants and children, improper brain development and subsequent mental retardation, poor metabolism, a lack of collagen production, a weak immune system, high serum cholesterol, irritability, depression, and a general susceptibility to stress. Women who take birth control pills show evidence of a B6 deficiency, which usually leads to depression. The pill also seems to create a glucose tolerance problem in women, which can lead to gestational diabetes once the pill is stopped and pregnancy occurs. It is not yet known whether these problems are merely coincidence or have a cause-and-effect relationship, but they seem to be easily alleviated by adequate ingestion of pyridoxine. Pyridoxine may also control the nausea that usually accompanies pregnancy.

The RDA for pyridoxine is 1.8-2.2 mg, and for pregnant women it is 2.5 mg. However, because this vitamin is easily lost in cooking or food processing, and women usually do not get even the basic RDA, partial or total deficiencies are more common than with other B vitamins. Therefore, it is not enough merely to eat the foods—such as meats, whole grains and brewer's yeast—that supply B6. It is necessary to supplement food intake, and it is probably wise to achieve at least the pregnancy RDA even for women who are not pregnant. Furthermore, it is recommended that every woman consult her doctor during pregnancy to consider increasing her intake of pyridoxine. In fact, women should consider increasing their pyridoxine intake before they become pregnant because higher levels of B6 in mothers may result in higher birthweight babies. In some pregnancies—in fact, many normal ones—the requirements for pyridoxine may double or triple over the nonpregnant state. This has led to recommendations that the supplemental range be between 5 and 20 mg daily. This is still nontoxic, but a physician should be consulted if the RDA is to be exceeded by this amount. With pyridoxine, a little more is probably better than a little less; and with all its important functions for both mother and baby, it is better to be on the safe side.

One other beneficial aspect of pyridoxine should be of interest to any parent. Vitamin B6 is capable of stopping convulsions in infants and children, and it is also being used to calm hyperactive children. Pyridoxine raises the level of serotonin in the system. Serotonin is a neurotransmitter in the brain that has a calming effect on the body. This is not to suggest that pregnant women or mothers with hyperactive children should arbitrarily provide megadoses of pyridoxine. Pyridoxine requirements vary with age, growth rate, caloric intake, and protein intake. The more protein that is eaten, the more B6 is needed to metabolize that protein. However, any amount that exceeds the RDA should be taken under the guidance of a doctor.

Cobalamin (B12)

Benefits to Your Baby: Aids nervous system development and formation of red blood cells. Involved in protein metabolism.

Cobalamin is the only B vitamin that contains a metal, cobalt. It is because of this that B12 is the largest molecule of all the vitamins. Its metallic properties make it impossible to manufacture this vitamin synthetically. It must be provided by animal protein, such as liver and other organ meats, or growth in bacteria and moulds, much like penicillin. Cobalamin is essential in increasing the longevity of cell life and is involved in food metabolism. It is also necessary for the structure and function of the nervous system, the metabolism of folate (an especially important nutrient during pregnancy), and the synthesis of nucleic acid. Cobalamin cannot be absorbed by the body unless in the presence of a sugar-protein substance called the *intrinsic factor*. If this substance is lacking, a B12 deficiency results.

Some of the disorders related to B12 deficiency include anaemia (because of this vitamin's relationship to folate), fatigue, hypoglycaemia, insomnia, nervousness, susceptibility to stress, and weight problems. Other symptoms include the impaired functioning of the small intestine (absorption problems), a delay in blood clotting (which can be dangerous during delivery), and visual difficulties. These deficiency symptoms are remedied by the ingestion of adequate amounts of cobalamin in the presence of the intrinsic factor.

The RDA for pregnant women is 4 mcg (micrograms). As with the other B vitamins, cobalamin is water-soluble and easily lost during cooking or processing. Therefore, women must be certain to eat enough cheese, fish, milk, organ meats, eggs, and cottage cheese to ensure they are getting enough B12. If you do not eat these foods, you must take a supplement that includes cobalamin.

Pangamic Acid (B15)

Benefits to Your Baby: May work in prevention of heart disease. Lowers blood cholesterol levels.

Pangamic acid is considered the vitamin that improves endurance performances, whether that of a long-distance athlete or a woman going through prolonged labour. The reason for this is that pangamic acid is heavily involved in cell respiration and oxidation processes. More specifically, B15 tends to prevent hypoxia, which is an insufficient supply of oxygen to the tissues. The importance of this is obvious when you realize that the heart is a muscle that requires oxygen to function properly in much the same way as other muscles.

Pangamic acid is also involved in metabolic processes, including protein, fat, and sugar metabolism. The vitamin has some beneficial effect on ateroscelerosis and diabetes because it lowers high blood cholesterol levels, improves circulation, and regulates metabolism. The nervous system and the endocrine system also benefit from proper amounts of pangamic acid in the diet.

A pangamic acid deficiency can have extremely deleterious effects on you and your baby. Symptoms include asthma, atherosclerosis (hardening of the arteries), high cholesterol, emphysema, heart disease, headaches, impaired circulation, insomnia, nervous system and glandular disorders, and shortness of breath. All of these deficiency symptoms can affect either your or your baby at any time during pregnancy, labour, or delivery.

Foods high in pangamic acid include brewer's yeast, brown rice, seeds, whole grains, and organ meats. Unfortunately, it is difficult to gauge how much B15 women should receive daily because no RDA has been established. The difficulty is increased because pregnant women require more of every other B vitamin than nonpregnant women.

Some clinical trials have shown that 2.5 to 10 mg daily of pangamic acid was completely nontoxic. In fact, there are some estimates that you would have to take more than 100,000 times these amounts before experiencing any possible side effects. Thus, in addition to all the beneficial effects of vitamin B15, we can add that it is relatively nontoxic, as are all the other B vitamins.

Biotin

Benefits to Your Baby: Prevents muscle cramping and soreness. Aids muscular development and motor control. May prevent cot death.

Biotin is a unique vitamin within the B complex in that it promotes the utilization of all the other B vitamins. It also helps regulate cell growth, assists in the oxidation and production of fatty acids in the body, aids in carbohydrate metabolism, improves the function of the thyroid and adrenal glands, and is a major factor in the body's production of energy.

Biotin is found in many of the same foods as the other B vitamins, and also in egg yolks, cauliflower, and mushrooms. Biotin deficiencies are rare, but they are manifested in specific symptoms. A biotin deficiency can occur if a woman eats too many egg whites. There is a substance in the egg white called avidin that binds with the biotin and renders it unavailable. The result is symptoms such as depression, dermatitis, insomnia, leg cramps, muscular pain and weakness, an impaired immune system with an increased susceptibility to stress, and a poor appetite. Biotin deficiencies have also been implicated in Sudden Infant Death Syndrome (SIDS).

All of these symptoms can have an effect on your pregnancy. The weaker you are, the less able you are to provide the foetus with everything it needs. The best way for you to receive adequate amounts of biotin, besides eating foods rich in this vitamin, is to supplement your dietary intake. The RDA of biotin for pregnant women should exceed the normal adult RDA of 300 mcg. However, ingestion of more than 500 mcg daily should not be undertaken without a physician's supervision. Remember that this range of 300–500 mcg is merely a recommendation. It is important to be aware that pregnant women have lower biotin levels than other adults, and these levels continue to decrease as the pregnancy progresses.

Choline

Benefits to Your Baby: Essential for healthy liver. Aids in circulatory system functions and memory development.

Choline's status as a vitamin is still controversial, but it is included here as part of the vitamin B complex because it occurs naturally with so many of the other B vitamins. Choline together with inositol (another B vitamin) are the basic components of lecithin. The primary function of choline is to prevent fat accumulation in the liver and to move fats in and out of cells. This may have positive effects on the body's ability to ward off heart disease and possibly cancer. Other functions of the vitamin include assisting in basic metabolism, nerve transmissions and memory development, and, as a component of lecithin, choline is essential for the health of the liver and the kidneys.

There are many symptoms associated with an inadequate supply of choline in the body. The ones relevant to pregnant women include atherosclerosis, bleeding stomach ulcers, high serum cholesterol, constipation, dizziness, high blood pressure, hypoglycemia, impaired liver and kidney function, insomnia, and various forms of heart disease. These symptoms can be prevented by adequate intake of choline, but there is no RDA for this vitamin. However, most diets provide up to 600 mg of choline daily. Pregnant women should try to take in somewhat more choline, up to 1,000 mg daily. The best food sources for this vitamin are brewer's yeast, fish, legumes, organ meats, lecithin, wheat germ, and egg yolks. Also, the body can make choline from the amino acid methionine when methionine interacts with B12 and folic acid (folate).

Folic Acid (Folate; Folacin)

Benefits to Your Baby: Works with iron to prevent anaemia. Needed for haemoglobin synthesis. Involved in synthesis of DNA and RNA. Involved in amino acid synthesis.

Folic acid is important to a variety of bodily functions. Its importance is magnified during pregnancy because it combines with iron to prevent anaemia.

Folic acid is also necessary for the synthesis of DNA and RNA and the subsequent cell reproduction. Folic acid functions as a coenzyme, along with B12 and vitamin C, in the breakdown and utilization of protein. The vitamin is necessary for proper brain function, improving both mental activity and emotional health. Finally, folic acid helps regulate the appetite and metabolic processes.

The primary function of folic acid is in the formation of red blood cells. Folic acid is the carbon carrier in haeme, the iron-containing protein that is found in red blood cells. A folic acid deficiency will result in anaemia, with a subsequent impairment of the immune system. The most observable evidence of this deficiency occurs in body systems that depend upon the rapid reproduction of new cells. Some of these systems are the bone marrow, fingernails and hair. Other deficiency symptoms include poor growth, gastrointestinal disturbances (which means a further decrease of folic acid in the body), metabolic disturbances, depression, general weakness, irritability, mental problems, and neurological changes.

About 25 percent of healthy pregnant women have

marginal to low serum folate levels. One reason is that there are increased demands for this vitamin, especially during the last 3 months of pregnancy. Another reason is that there is increased excretion of the vitamin during pregnancy. Pregnant women who have low folate levels face a double-edged sword. First, folic acid deficiency can lead to anaemia and it may also lead to toxemia, which is the premature separation of the placenta from the wall of the uterus. Second, women with this problem have a tendency to deliver low-birthweight or malformed babies. Children of low-folate mothers also have less resistance to disease and may evidence a slowdown in their mental and physical development.

The best preventative measure is to ensure that you take in adequate amounts of folic acid before you become pregnant. Then continue eating foods that contain folic acid, such as vegetables, dairy products, whole grains, brewer's yeast, and organ meats, and supplement your diet with folic acid. The RDA for pregnant women is 800 mcg, while for nonpregnant women, it is 400 mcg. It is imperative that a nonpregnant woman receive at least these minimal amounts daily because if she becomes pregnant when she is folate deficient, damage may be done to the foetus early in its life. Low-folate mothers who suffer from anaemia may not be able to correct the problem with folate or iron supplements. One of the symptoms of folic acid deficiency is an absorption problem, and if the vitamin cannot be absorbed into the system, the deficiency perpetuates itself. Fortunately, more often than not, the body does absorb the folic acid and begins to correct the deficiency. Most, if not all, doctors agree that folic acid supplementation is necessary during pregnancy. This is especially true during the last 3 months, when the foetus places increased demands on the mother and the mother places increased demands on herself simply by carrying the foetus and preparing for labour and delivery. However, arbitrary supplementation is not recommended. Folic acid levels can be measured, and the exact amount that is necessary can be prescribed by your doctor.

Inositol

Benefits to Your Baby: Aids in development of nervous system and prevention of heart disease.

Inositol is a versatile B vitamin that is closely associated with biotin and choline. Inositol, like choline, is found in high concentrations in lecithin. Many of the major organs, such as the brain, heart, kidneys, and liver, benefit from adequate amounts of inositol. The primary functions of this vitamin are the metabolism of fats and their removal from the system to prevent heart disease, the reduction of blood cholesterol levels, an improvement in nerve conduction, and the protection of the liver, kidneys, and heart.

Deficiency symptoms related to inositol are rare simply because the body contains more of this vitamin than any other except niacin. If a deficiency were ever to occur, most of the symptoms would be related to the heart: hardening of the arteries, high cholesterol, and the development of heart disease. Some of the other symptoms include constipation, skin problems, and possibly obesity, which is a risk factor in both the pregnant and nonpregnant state.

Inositol is found in many of the same foods as the other B vitamins, plus blackstrap molasses, citrus fruits, milk, nuts, and vegetables. There is no established RDA for pregnant women. The recommendation is that inositol intake be similar to choline intake, and that is about 1,000 mg a day. Simply by adding lecithin to your diet you can guarantee that you will be getting enough choline and inositol.

Para-Aminobenzoic Acid (PABA)

Benefits to Your Baby: Maintains healthy skin. May deter aging and cancer process. Aids in the production of pantothenic acid.

PABA is probably best known for its sunscreen properties,

but it actually does serve a function as a B vitamin. PABA stimulates intestinal bacteria to produce folic acid, which, in addition to all its beneficial effects on pregnancy, also aids in the production of pantothenic acid. This function of PABA further illustrates the synergistic workings of the B vitamins. Other functions of PABA include the breakdown and utilization of protein, the formation of red blood cells, the maintenance of healthy skin, and hair pigmentation. The role of PABA in pregnancy has not been well established and can only be extrapolated from the benefits mentioned above.

Deficiency symptoms related to PABA are rare, but when they do occur they mirror some of the problems that are common in pregnancy. These include constipation, depression, digestive disorders, fatigue, headaches, irritability, stress reactions, and skin disorders. There is speculation that PABA is related to the greying of hair, but no conclusive evidence has been produced.

There is no RDA for PABA, but up to 30 mg daily has been shown to have no harmful effects. Ingestion of more than this amount should be reserved for therapeutic purposes, and then taken only under the guidance of a doctor. An important point to remember about PABA is that it should not be taken with sulphur drugs because they render each other useless.

Vitamin C (Ascorbic Acid)

Benefits to Your Baby: Aids in tissue formation and maintains integrity of immune system. "Cement" in connective and vascular tissues. Increases iron absorption.

Vitamin C is probably the most well known of the vitamins. The claims for its beneficial effects are endless, from preventing the common cold to curing heart disease and cancer. No such claims are made here. Rather, vitamin C is described as it is known to function in the body.

Vitamin C is unstable and sensitive to oxygen. That is

why you hear people say that when orange juice is exposed to air, much of the vitamin C is destroyed. The same is also said about supplements. The vitamin is also sensitive to light and heat. Therefore, we have to be careful how we get our vitamin C and if we are actually getting enough on a daily basis.

The primary function of vitamin C is the formation and maintenance of collagen, which is connective tissue. Other functions include aiding in wound and burn healing, the formation of red blood cells, the prevention of haemorrhaging, and the strengthening of the immune system. Vitamin C also plays an interactive role with other nutrients. It protects many of the B complex vitamins from oxidation, which is why vitamin C is classified as an antioxidant. The vitamin helps in the absorption of iron, and assists in the conversion of folic acid to its active form, folinic acid. Both of these functions are vitally important during pregnancy, especially in the treatment or prevention of anaemia. Vitamin C is also found in large quantities in the adrenal glands, where it is used to help the body combat stress. Finally, vitamin C plays a role in the metabolism of several amino acids.

There has been extreme interest in the role vitamin C plays in the prevention of heart disease. Vitamin C has been shown to lower both cholesterol and triglyceride levels while increasing the level of HDL (high-density lipoprotein) in the blood. HDL is the good cholesterol, and higher levels are known to be a deterrent to heart disease. Vitamin C is also capable of slowing down the blood-clotting process, and these clots are one of the causes of cardiovascular disease. If you're wondering whether or not large doses of vitamin C will prevent heart disease, the answer is no. However, vitamin C will contribute to the prevention of heart disease when combined with prudent living habits.

It is rare today to see a vitamin C deficiency, but the most well-known deficiency disease is scurvy. Some of the symptoms associated with scurvy include haemorrhaging, delayed wound healing, broken bones, generalized swelling, and inflammation of the gums. Other deficiency symptoms related to vitamin C are anaemia, general fatigue and weakness, irritability, easy bruising and bleeding, pain in the joints that could lead to arthritis or bursitis, depression, and possible neurological disturbances. Infants who have a vitamin C deficiency show many of these latter symptoms, most of the scurvy symptoms, plus impaired growth and development. Furthermore, the deficiency can be transferred from the mother to the foetus. If the mother is not receiving enough vitamin C, bone and tissue formation in the foetus will be abnormal, and other systems in the foetus will not develop properly.

The importance of vitamin C to a pregnant woman is magnified by the fact that maternal levels of the vitamin progressively decline throughout the pregnancy. In fact, blood levels at full-term are often one-half of what they were at midpregnancy. Additionally, the foetal requirement of vitamin C is so high that mothers must be sure they continuously replenish their supply. It is not uncommon for a large portion of the maternal vitamin C to be concentrated in the placenta, thereby placing the foetal levels at 50 percent or more above maternal levels.

The RDA for vitamin C is currently 60 mg for nonpregnant women. The RDA for pregnant women is 80 mg. Neither of these doses is exceptionally high when compared to recommendations that you should take one, two, even five thousand milligrams of vitamin C a day for optimum health. While these large doses may not be harmful to a healthy, nonpregnant woman, pregnant women must be cautioned about ingesting megadoses of vitamin C. Even though there are no defined toxicity levels, high intake of vitamin C during pregnancy may have adverse effects on foetal development. Furthermore, an infant who adapts and becomes accustomed to high levels of vitamin C during the gestational period will probably suffer from an acute deficiency that may be harmful when the maternal supply is stopped at birth. Therefore, the recommendation is to remain within the RDA limits by eating fresh fruits and vegetables, and supplementing when necessary.

Vitamin D

Benefits to Your Baby: Aids absorption of calcium and phosphorus. Helps build strong bones and teeth.

Vitamin D is a fat-soluble vitamin that has been called the sunshine vitamin. This is because the sun's ultraviolet rays activate a form of cholesterol present in the skin and convert it to vitamin D. Therefore, we can get our supply of vitamin D either from exposure to sunlight or through our diet. Vitamin D has also been called the "children's vitamin" because it helps with their growth and development.

Vitamin D's main role is to help the body absorb calcium and phosphorus for the formation of bones and cartilage. It is also important to the development of strong teeth. In fact, any process in the body that requires calcium also requires vitamin D. This includes the function of the heart and nervous system, the synthesis of enzymes in the body's mucous membranes, where calcium is transported, and the normal clotting of blood. Vitamin D best performs its role when it is taken with vitamin A, as the two have a positive interactive effect.

When a woman suffers from a vitamin D deficiency, blood levels of the vitamin and of calcium will drop. The body will then retrieve calcium from the bones, causing a condition known as osteomalacia, or soft bones. Children who are deficient in vitamin D develop a condition called rickets. This occurs when calcium and phosphorus are not deposited in the cartilage and the bones swell with cartilage at the ends and are soft and malformed in the middle. Also, tooth enamel will develop in a thin and irregular fashion. Basically, this means that there is faulty mineralization of the body's bony structures. The softness of the bones leads to an inability to bear weight, which results in skeletal malformations these include a softening of the skull, bowing of the legs, excessive spinal curvature, enlargement of the wrist, knee, and ankle joints, and poorly developed muscles.

Children with a vitamin D deficiency are nervous, irritable, restless, begin to crawl late, walk late, have a soft skull, develop bone malformations and neuromuscular problems, and possibly go into spasms. These symptoms can all be prevented by ensuring that both you and your baby receive enough vitamin D every day.

The RDA for vitamin D is 400-600 IU for pregnant women. This can readily be obtained from foods rich in vitamin D, such as egg yolks, cod liver oil, organ meats, milk, tuna, or salmon. Also, remember that sunlight is an excellent source of vitamin D. If you are going to take vitamin D supplements, they should be taken only after a meal. Because the vitamin is fat-soluble, you should have food in your system to help with its storage and utilization. Furthermore, vitamin D in large doses can be toxic. Toxicity symptoms include high blood levels of calcium and phosphorus, excessive excretion of calcium in the urine, which leads to calcification of the soft tissues of the kidneys (hypercalcemia), loss of appetite, nausea, vomiting, muscular weakness, dizziness, and calcification of the soft tissues of the heart, lungs, and blood vessels.

Vitamin E (Tocopherol)

Benefits to Your Baby: Enhances absorption of vitamin A. Aids tissue growth, cell wall development, circulation, and red blood cell integrity.

Vitamin E is a fat-soluble vitamin that has had many nicknames. It has been called the 'sex vitamin, the "anti-aging vitamin" and the "heart vitamin".' These names stem from the apparent benefits that vitamin E provides.

The primary role of vitamin E is as an antioxidant, which means it prevents the oxidation of substances in the body. For example, vitamin E prevents saturated fatty acids and vitamin A from breaking down and combining with other substances in the body that may prove harmful. If these breakdowns are allowed to occur, substances known as free radicals are created. Free radicals are destructive molecules that can cause cancer, unwanted blood clots, and damage to the structure of DNA. The importance of vitamin E's role is even more apparent when you consider that every cell requires fat to function, either for protection or for energy.

The secondary functions of vitamin E relate to cellular metabolism and respiration. Vitamin E combines with oxygen so that red blood cells can remain fully supplied with oxygenated blood. This improves the function of the heart and circulatory system. The vitamin also enables muscles and nerves to function longer with less oxygen, thereby increasing endurance. This is especially important to you during labour and delivery.

Vitamin E has still more functions. They include prevention of blood clots, dilation of blood vessels for better circulation, possible slowing of the aging process, allowance for great storage of vitamin A and therefore a reduction in its requirement, promotion of wound healing and tissue growth, stimulation of urine excretion, pollution protection in the lungs, relief from headaches, removal of cholesterol from the artery walls, and a reduction in blood pressure. Some of the beneficial effects of vitamin E, such as improved circulation, endurance, and muscular function, are probably the reason people believed it improved their sex lives. The fact is that the combination of vitamin E's beneficial effects leads to an improvement in the functioning of most of the body's systems, and the reproductive system is just one of them.

Deficiency symptoms associated with vitamin E include degeneration of the sex organs in males, a delay in the onset of puberty in adolescents, diminished function of the thyroid gland, possible muscular degeneration, and a reduction in the survival time and production of red blood cells. It is also possible that a vitamin E deficiency can have a degenerative effect on the brain and spinal cord of children. Infants also may suffer from a vitamin E deficiency, especially since they have less than one-fifth the blood levels their mothers have. Premature babies show even lower concentrations than full-term infants. The result is a form of anaemia caused by an increased rate of destruction of red blood cells. The mistake often made in the treatment of this condition is that iron supplements or injections are given without vitamin E supplementation. The result is an aggravation of the anaemic reaction.

One other point about vitamin E and infants should be mentioned. Premature infants are usually given oxygen at birth to help them breathe. However, this can have a harmful effect because their lung tissue can start oxidizing and breaking down. Currently, the recommended treatment in this instance, and the one supported by most doctors, is supplementation of vitamin E before administering oxygen. This is either done by injection or orally. The infant's lungs are then protected.

Pregnant women should adhere to the RDA for vitamin E, which is 15 IU. Since this is a fat-soluble vitamin, there can be toxic effects from large doses, such as an increase in blood pressure. Although toxicity is rare, any amounts above 15 IU a day should be approved by your doctor.

Vitamin E supplements are not always necessary, because this vitamin is readily available from the foods we eat. These include dark green vegetables, eggs, liver, wheat germ, vegetable oils, oatmeal, peanuts, and tomatoes. Remember, if you are going to use supplements, take them after a meal and in conjunction with vitamin A.

Vitamin F (Unsaturated Fatty Acids)

Benefits to Your Baby: Provide body's cells with protection and are used as source of energy.

Vitamin F is not truly a vitamin. It is more of a classification for unsaturated fatty acids. It is mentioned here because these fatty acids play a key role in cellular function. They provide cells with protection and are used as sources of energy. Every diet should include unsaturated fatty acids in a ratio of two to one over saturated fatty acids. We receive "vitamin F" from such foods as vegetable oils, wheat germ, and seeds.

Vitamin K (Menadione)

Benefits to Your Baby: Aids in blood clotting.

Vitamin K is a fat-soluble vitamin that can be manufactured by the body in the intestines. A diet that includes yogurt, acidophilus milk, and unsaturated fatty acids will allow the body to produce adequate amounts of this vitamin. The primary function of vitamin K is in the formation of prothrombin, a substance required for blood clotting. The vitamin is also involved in a chemical conversion process in which carbohydrates are converted into glycogen so they can be stored by the body. Finally, as with all fat-soluble vitamins, K can help with the proper functioning of the liver. The liver is responsible for supplying bile, which is necessary for the body to absorb the fat-soluble vitamins.

Although there is not specific RDA for vitamin K, it is believed that between 300 and 500 mcg is an adequate daily supply. Infants require 1-5 mg to prevent abnormal bleeding, which is the primary deficiency symptom associated with vitamin K. The body is unable to produce clots, and haemorrhaging can occur. Other symptoms include bruises, diarrhoea, and the possibility of an increased incidence of miscarriage. It is important for women to eat a diet that provides them with natural sources of vitamin K. These include green, leafy vegetables, blackstrap molasses, yogurt, oatmeal, egg yolks, fish liver oils, kelp, alfalfa, sunflower oil and other polyunsaturated oils. However, the best and most dependable supply comes from intestinal bacteria.

Since vitamin K is a fat-soluble vitamin, it can produce toxic effects when taken in high doses. Therapeutic doses of vitamin K have been given to women just before labour to prevent haemorrhaging, but this is always under a doctor's direction. Too much K at other times can make you anaemic because red blood cells are broken down and destroyed. Also, infants can overdose on vitamin K when their mothers take too much of this vitamin. Granules form in the infant's red blood cells that damage the haemoglobin.

Bioflavonoids (Vitamin P)

Benefits to Your Baby: Prevents excess bleeding. Enhances absorption of vitamin C.

Bioflavonoids are water-soluble vitamins that are essential for the proper absorption and utilization of vitamin C. The bioflavonoids are citrin, flavonals, flavones, hesperidin, and rutin. Basically, these substances minimize the body's tendency to bruise, and strengthen the walls of the blood vessels, thereby preventing haemorrhaging.

There is no RDA for bioflavonoids and they are presumed nontoxic. The bioflavonoids enhance the functional utility of vitamin C. Thus, beneficial effects can be seen in the circulatory system, the immune system, the skeleton system, and in the body's ability to withstand stress. A specific benefit to pregnant women is that bioflavonoids strengthen capillary walls and reduce or prevent excessive bleeding.

Minerals

Most people are very familiar with vitamins and the way they can benefit the body. Unfortunately, the same level of familiarity does not hold true for minerals. Yet minerals are as important to life and normal human functioning as are vitamins, and in some cases, minerals are even more important. The basic premise with regard to minerals is that they are so vital to creating health and well-being that vitamins cannot function properly without them.

Approximately 25 minerals are necessary for proper bodily functions. Nineteen of these are considered essential; that is, the body must have them in adequate supply in order for each cell to perform its work. Some of these essential minerals, also called *macrominerals* because they are required in relatively large amounts, include calcium, phosphorus, potassium, sodium, chlorine, and magnesium. Other minerals are considered *trace elements* because they are required in small amounts. These trace elements include iron, zinc, solinium, iodine, and copper, as well as several others.

In contrast to vitamins, which are organic, minerals are inorganic compounds. Minerals are directly responsible for the body's functions of growth, development, and maintenance. This is again in direct contrast to vitamins, which *aid* the various organs and systems in carrying out their functions. Since minerals help create the environment in which vitamins perform their work, it is easy to see the importance of the relationship between the two. That is why no one should ever take a multivitamin supplement without take a multimineral supplement. Vitamins and minerals work synergistically and they must be taken together for maximum benefit.

It was once believe that no person could ever suffer from any type of mineral deficiency because minerals are in such abundant supply in nature. However, chemicals and food processing techniques tend to rob food of important minerals. Research has shown that eating a diet high in refined and processed foods can lead to a variety of mineral deficiencies. Continued eating along these lines can lead to even more serious diseases such as goitre (thyroid) and anaemia. The other side of the coin also poses a problem. While minerals are necessary for good health and well-being, too much of a mineral can also lead to illness. A person who takes too much of a particular mineral upsets the delicate balance required between other minerals and vitamins for the body's proper functioning. Therefore, as with vitamins, no one, especially pregnant women, should supplement their diet with a multimineral tablet unless under the supervision of her doctor.

Minerals possess tremendous qualities as aids to proper bodily functions. They can help provide a person with energy, make wounds heal faster, prevent a variety of pregnancy problems, and assist in the proper growth and development of the foetus. All these functions will be described in the next section of this chapter. Each important mineral is presented along with its functions, its food sources, the beneficial effects it has on the body, and its relationship to pregnancy. It is important to remember that minerals, like vitamins, are necessary for good health, but they can only work well when taken in the correct amounts.

Calcium

Benefits to Your Baby: Builds bones and teeth. Aids in muscle contraction, blood clotting, and regulation of heartbeat. Regulates use of other minerals in the body. Foetal requirements increase in last 3 months.

Calcium is the most abundant mineral in the body. It is the main structural mineral, as 99 percent of the body's calcium is in the bones and teeth. It is not as if the calcium is deposited in these structures permanently. Rather, they serve as calcium reservoirs for the body to draw upon. There is a constant exchange of this mineral among the bones, body fluids, and soft tissues. If calcium exceeds supply, the body draws upon its calcium stores to maintain adequate blood levels. The problem is that the calcium that is lost from the bones must be replaced, or it is lost forever. The other one percent of calcium is involved in the blood-clotting process, nerve and muscle function, parathyroid hormone function, metabolism of vitamin D, and the function of the heart.

Calcium's main job is to work with phosphorus to build

and maintain strong bones and teeth. In fact, calcium and phosphorous must occur together so that both may function properly. The ratio of calcium to phosphorus in the body is 2.5 to 1, but current recommendations are that people should receive the same amount of calcium and phosphorus each day. Several other vitamins and minerals are required for calcium to function properly. These are magnesium, vitamin A, C, D, and possibly E. All of them should be taken with calcium to improve the absorption process. Usually, only 20 to 30 percent of ingested calcium is absorbed by the body. We excrete about 100-200 mg of calcium in the urine and another 125-180 mg in the faeces daily.

If calcium supply does not meet demand, other important functions of calcium will be hindered. Calcium regulates the heartbeat, helps control the contraction and relaxation of the heart muscle, aids in blood clotting, and prevents the accumulation of too much acid in the blood. In fact, calcium requires acid in the digestive system to be absorbed, and if there is not enough acid, calcium won't dissolve and deposits will form. When this occurs in the joints, the result is a limited range of movement and extreme pain. If calcium deposits occur in the circulatory system, the results can be disastrous: atherosclerosis or a heart attack.

Some of the other functions of calcium include its role in muscle growth, muscle contraction, nerve transmission, the utilization of iron, and the passage of nutrients through cell walls. These functions are as important as building strong bones and teeth and regulating the heart. They are just not as well publicized.

Calcium plays an especially important role in pregnancy. All of the mineral's functions mentioned above are vital to your health, well-being, and strength during the entire term. The growth and development function of calcium becomes extremely important during the last 3 months. You deposit between 200 and 300 mg of calcium daily in the skeleton of the foetus. If you are not receiving an adequate daily supply, the foetus will extract the calcium from your bones. If the calcium is not replaced, the bone health of both you and your baby will suffer. The same sequence of events can occur if you are breast-feeding. Breast milk contains between 250 and 500 mg of calcium each day, and if this is not replaced, the mineral will be drawn from your bones.

Deficiency symptoms include muscle spasms and convulsions, irregular heartbeats, nervousness, bone malformations in children, and osteomalacia or osteoporosis (brittle bones). Most of these deficiencies are rare, but osteoporosis is common among middle-aged and elderly women. The simple reason is that their calcium demands have exceeded their supplies, and the reserves have not been replenished.

The RDA for calcium is 800-1,200 mg, with pregnant women requiring 1,200-1,600 mg. There is a strong possibility that this RDA level is too low because of all the important ways in which the body uses calcium. However, if you are planning to exceed these levels, consult your doctor. Too much calcium can cause serious disease symptoms, such as calcium deposits in the heart, circulatory system, kidneys, muscles, joints, and other areas of the body. Excess calcium also leads to a condition known as hypercalcemia, which is simply too much calcium in the blood without enough places to use it. The result can be kidney stones.

The best sources of calcium are milk and dairy products. The mineral can also be found in molasses, almonds, and liver. The number of foods that supply adequate amounts of calcium is obviously small. Therefore, it is often best to consider supplementing dietary intake with some sort of tablet. This is especially true if you are not eating properly as your term progresses. A rule of thumb regarding calcium is that we need, at a minimum, the equivalent of 2 pints of milk a day, every day of our lives.

Chromium

Benefits to Your Baby: Aids in glucose regulation and synthesis of fatty acids.

Chromium is an essential mineral in the body. Its primary function is to work with insulin to metabolize sugar. Chromium is an active ingredient in the glucose tolerance factor (GTF), which is also made up of niacin and amino acids. The GTF is responsible not only for the metabolism of glucose but also the synthesis of fatty acids and cholesterol. Basically, chromium aids the body in developing its energy supply. Some other functions of chromium include synthesis of proteins, DNA, and RNA.

Adequate amounts of chromium in the system prevent hypoglycemia (too little sugar) and diabetes (too much sugar, too little insulin). Chromium deficiencies can lead to either of these conditions, as well as increased cholesterol levels in the blood and the production of plaque. There may also be depressed growth rates and severe glucose intolerance. Pregnant women are more susceptible to deficiencies of this mineral because the developing foetus requires so much.

There is no specific RDA for chromium, but most people receive between 80 and 100 mcg daily. The problem is that chromium is difficult to absorb, and with no RDA, we can never be sure we are getting enough. To be on the safe side, it is best to take in .05–.2 mg of chromium each day, especially when you are pregnant. There is no known toxicity for chromium because the body effectively eliminates excessive amounts. The best food sources of chromium are brewer's yeast, clams, corn oil, liver, blackstrap molasses, cheese, and whole grains.

Copper

Benefits to Your Baby: Assists in formation of red blood cells. Forms protective myelin sheath around nerves. Aids in energy metabolism.

Copper is one of the most important trace minerals in the

body. It assists in the formation of haemoglobin and red blood cells by facilitating iron absorption. It also aids in the generation of cellular energy, the linking of collagen, the formation of melanin (pigmentation) and elastin, and the development of the myelin sheath that covers nerve fibres. It also contributes to the sense of taste. Some other functions of this vital mineral include converting the amino acid tyrosine into a dark pigment that colours the hair and skin, aiding in the healing process, oxidizing vitamin C and working with it to form elastin, producing RNA, and developing and maintaining proper bone formation.

True copper deficiencies are rare, but there are specific symptoms associated with a deficiency. These include abnormal pigmentation, defects in the elastic tissue of the blood vessels, anaemia, general weakness, impaired respiration, skin sores, improper development of bones and nerves, and a loss of taste. Conversely, there are also toxic symptoms associated with an overdose of copper. Too much copper can lead to serious physical and mental illness, heart attacks, high blood pressure, toxemia in pregnancy, premenstrual tension, depression, insomnia, and functional hypoglycaemia. Pregnant women tend to have high copper levels, which causes a decrease in iron and a deficiency of molybdenum. In fact, certain anaemic conditions that are not helped by supplemental iron may be due to elevated copper levels. Furthermore, because copper levels do rise throughout pregnancy, it can take up to three months for them to return to normal after delivery. This may partly account for post-partum depression.

The RDA for copper is 2-4 mg for pregnant women, and the best food sources include legumes, nuts, seafood, organ meats, raisins, molasses, mushrooms, chocolate, bone meal, and soya beans. When your diet does not regularly include these foods, then supplementation is necessary. You must receive adequate amounts of copper, not only for yourself but to help your baby form haemoglobin and to prevent edaema and possible nutritional disorders.

Fluorine

Benefits to Your Baby: Aids in strengthening bones and teeth. Enhances calcium utilization. Protects against magnesium deficiency.

Fluorine is by far the most controversial of all the vitamins and minerals. This is because it is the only nutrient that is added to public water supplies. The debate still rages as to whether or not this supplement actually helps fight cavities. The main function of fluorine is to help build strong bones and teeth by improving the absorption of calcium. Fluorine also reduces the formation of acid in the mouth, thereby preventing tooth decay. When fluorine is available during tooth development, it becomes part of the mineral structure of the teeth. The same process probably occurs in bone development.

Fluoridated water provides the best supply of this mineral, and if you drink 6-8 glasses of water each day, you will receive an adequate supply of fluorine. The RDA for pregnant women is 1.5-4 mg, and it comes from water, seafood, cheese, meat, apples, eggs, and milk. Deficiencies of fluorine are rare, but it is possible to receive too much fluorine. Toxic symptoms include depressed growth, calcification of the ligaments and tendons, and degenerative changes in the kidneys, heart, liver, adrenal glands, and nervous system. People may also suffer allergic reactions to too much fluorine, such as dermatitis, acne, hives, excessive thirst, and headaches.

Iodine

Benefits to Your Baby: Controls rate of energy usage. Aids in the function of the thyroid. Promotes growth and development.

Iodine is a trace mineral that is converted into iodide in the body. The primary purpose of this mineral is to aid in the development and function of the thyroid gland and regulate the production of thyroxin. Thyroxin is the hormone that regulates the metabolic rate of the body.

Other functions of iodine include regulating the production of energy, promoting growth and development, and helping the body "burn" excess fat. Iodine, through its role in the thyroid gland, also influences mental skills, speech, and the condition of the hair, skin, teeth, and nails. Other bodily processes, such as the conversion of carotene to vitamin A, the absorption of carbohydrates from the intestines, and the synthesis of protein, all occur more easily when the thyroid is functioning effectively.

The importance of iodine is demonstrated when there is a deficiency. The most common and well-known deficiency symptom is goitre. Goitre occurs when iodine supplies are diminished and the thyroid gland tries to compensate by producing more thyroxin. The gland becomes enlarged and congested. When a pregnant woman has goitre, or simply an iodine deficiency, her developing foetus runs the risk of being born physically and mentally retarded. This condition is known as cretinism. Iodine treatment can reverse this condition, but treatment must be started soon after birth.

There are other symptoms associated with a lack of iodine. These include hardening of the arteries, possible obesity due to a sluggish metabolism, decreased mental abilities, dry hair, heart palpitations and rapid pulse, tremor, irritability, nervousness, and restlessness. However, iodine deficiency in this country is rare. This is because iodine is added to salt and is abundant in seafood.

There is an RDA of 100-150 mcg for iodine, with a possible increase to 200 mcg in certain pregnancies. Although iodine toxicity is rare through food ingestion, toxicity can occur when overdoses of this mineral are taken as a supplement or a drug. The toxic symptoms are similar to the deficiency symptoms. Pregnant women should never arbitrarily supplement their food with iodine. Unsupervised supplementation can create special problems for women who have an undetected metabolic defect. This may cause them to react adversely when other women would respond normally to similar doses of the mineral. Two possible reactions could be an increased metabolism and interference with the iodine-thyroid gland-thyroxine production system.

Iron

Benefits to Your Baby: Foetal requirements increase tenfold during last six weeks of pregnancy. Combines with protein to form haemoglobin and prevents anaemia. Helps mother to sustain energy levels.

Iron is probably the mineral most associated with pregnancy. This is because iron is primarily responsible for the manufacture of haemoglobin, the oxygen-carrying protein in the blood. When there is not enough iron present, the result is anaemia.

Iron is needed by and is present in every cell in the body, combined with protein. In addition to its role in the production of haemoglobin, iron is also necessary for the formation of myoglobin. Myoglobin is the receptor and storage point for oxygen in the muscles, and its transfer of oxygen to the muscle cells permits contraction and movement. The other important function of iron is to maintain the health and integrity of red blood cells. High-quality blood provides superior nourishment to all cells, and this builds immunity to stress and disease.

The importance of iron to you and your baby cannot be overestimated. Anaemia is a reduction in the oxygen-carrying capacity of the blood, and the visible symptoms are pallor, fatigue, weakness, headaches, palpitations, laboured breathing during exercise or mild exertion, constipation, and brittle nails. Unfortunately, iron deficiency is often diagnosed when the deficiency is one of vitamin B6 and zinc, which mimics iron deficiencies. The best way to be certain that an iron deficiency exists is to measure serum iron levels rather than haemoglobin. The best way to prevent an iron deficiency is to be certain the vitamins and minerals that iron works best with are always in adequate supply. These nutrients include vitamins B6 and B12, vitamin C, copper, folic acid (of primary importance), and zinc.

The RDA of iron for nonpregnant women is about 18 mg, and this is because the body only absorbs about one-tenth of the iron it takes in. The requirements for a pregnant woman are substantially higher, you may need to increase your intake by three to four times the RDA, especially during the last 3 months. This means that the RDA can rise to as much as 60 mg by the end of the term. The reason for this is that blood volume increases by 50 percent during pregnancy, thereby increasing the need for haemoglobin. Additionally, the foetal requirements for iron increase as the term nears its end. The foetus can store enough iron in its liver during the last six weeks of pregnancy to supplement its need for the first three to six months of life. This should not be surprising, since breast milk and formula only partially fulfill the iron requirements of a newborn.

There are times when both you and your baby will need an additional supply of iron. These include periods of rapid growth, such as the last 3 months of pregnancy, and during menstruation or when there is any loss of blood. While foods that are rich in iron, such as blackstrap molasses, eggs, fish, liver, poultry, wheat-germ, apples, beans, oysters, almonds, and walnuts should be eaten, because they can often supply the RDA, many doctors recommend iron supplements during pregnancy. It has been mentioned several times in this book that supplementation should never be undertaken without a doctor's guidance. This is especially true in the case of iron. The importance of this mineral mandates that supplementary dosages be prescribed that are specific to each individual, especially during pregnancy. This recommendation is made to guarantee the effectiveness of iron utilization rather than to guard against toxicity. Iron toxicity is rare because the body will usually excrete iron. However, megadoses of iron are definitely not recommended for anyone.

Magnesium

Benefits to Your Baby: Aids in calcium functions. Coenzyme in energy and protein metabolism. Essential in cellular metabolism, muscle actions, and tissue growth. Can prevent formation of blood clots in the heart.

Magnesium is an essential mineral whose importance is not generally known. This mineral makes up .05 percent of total body weight, with most of it concentrated in the bones, along with calcium and phosphorus. A smaller amount of magnesium is found in the body's soft tissues and fluids. This would lead to the conclusion that magnesium is important for the growth, development, and function of the skeletal system. This is true, but the primary function of this mineral is to regulate cell metabolism and growth. Magnesium is so central to the life of a cell that almost all chemical reactions in the body require magnesium.

Magnesium aids in the production of energy and activates the enzymes necessary for the metabolism of carbohydrates and amino acids. The balance of magnesium and calcium in muscle cells regulates the contraction of muscles along with the transmissions in the nervous system.

Magnesium also plays other roles in the body together with several vitamins and minerals. Magnesium helps promote the absorption and metabolism of calcium, phosphorus, potassium, and sodium. These are all minerals involved in muscular contraction and movement. Magnesium also enables the body to better utilize the B complex vitamins and vitamins C and E. The combination of all these effects may lead to a role for magnesium in the regulation of body temperature.

Magnesium's contributions to pregnant women and their foetuses are magnified because the mineral is involved in so many vital functions. Its role in cellular and energy metabolism, neuromuscular function, heart function, bone growth and development, soft tissue growth, and the possible regulation of body temperature makes this mineral essential for a healthy pregnancy, labour, delivery, and growth of the infant.

Some of the deficiency symptoms include increased nervous system transmission, which leads to muscular irritability; increased speed of muscular contractions, improper calcium metabolism, leading to bone deformities, degeneration of the kidneys, skin, teeth, skeletal and cardiac muscles, and decreased blood levels of calcium and potassium, which leads to increased levels of sodium, resulting in edaema (swelling). More severe symptoms, such as stupor, coma, and psychotic behaviour, can also occur. Children who suffer from a magnesium deficiency will evidence a loss of appetite, retarded growth and development, apathy, hallucinations, irritability, confusion, weakness, tremors, twitches, apnea (breathing stops), and a rapid pulse. It is even possible that a connection may exist between a magnesium deficiency and sudden infant death syndrome (cot death).

The RDA of magnesium for pregnant women is 450 mg. This may not seem high, but the typical western diet only provides about 120 mg of magnesium per 1,000 calories ingested. Therefore, if you consume 2,200-2,500 calories a day, you may not be getting enough magnesium to satisfy even the RDA. Obviously, supplementation will be needed. Magnesium is readily available in many common foods, such as bran, honey, green vegetables, nuts, seafood, whole grains, milk, corn, and apples. However, the absorption of this mineral is heavily dependent upon the availability of calcium, phosphorus, vitamin D, lactose (milk sugar), parathyroid hormone, and the rate of water absorption in the body. If there is a deficiency in any of these, the amount of magnesium in the body will be further deweaked. Magnesium toxicity is rare because the intestines regulate the body's absorption of this mineral. However, if an overdose were to occur, it would probably have a laxative effect. This may be carried further to states of lethargy, drowsiness, and even anaesthesia. Therefore, it is imperative that any supplementation of magnesium be done under a doctor's guidance.

One other point must be made about magnesium. The interrelationship between magnesium and calcium is such that there must always be a balance in blood levels of these minerals. If calcium levels are high, magnesium levels must also be high. This is especially true of the heart. A high level of calcium and a lower level of magnesium could result in calcium deposits in the heart, kidneys, and blood vessels, which could lead to a heart attack or other forms of coronary artery disease. A proper amount of magnesium in the system can prevent the formation of blood clots in the heart, as well as protecting the body against high levels of cholesterol.

Manganese

Benefits to Your Baby: Aids in production of insulin and prevention of gestational diabetes. Involved in production of milk.

Manganese is an essential trace mineral that is present in all human tissue. It acts as a cofactor in activating numerous enzyme systems. Manganese is involved in the synthesis of protein, DNA, RNA, cartilaginous tissue, fatty acids, and cholesterol. Manganese also aids in the utilization of choline, and activates enzymes that are needed for the utilization of biotin, thiamine, and ascorbic acid. The mineral plays a role in normal skeletal development, may have some involvement in the formation of blood, aids in the production of milk and urea (a part of the urine), maintains sex hormone production, helps nourish the nerves and the brain, is essential for the production of thyroxin, and has an important role in the production and utilization of insulin.

Insulin is involved with sugar metabolism and therefore energy production. Insulin is also the hormone that is involved in diabetes (too little sugar in the blood or too much insulin). Since many women contract gestational diabetes, it is possible they may be suffering from a mild manganese deficiency. Similarly, if breast milk production is poor, there may be low levels of this mineral in the blood.

Other symptoms of a manganese deficiency include atherosclerosis (hardening of the arteries), muscle coordination failure, breathing problems, allergies, weight loss, determatitis, nausea, paralysis, convulsions, blindness and deafness in infants, dizziness and hearing loss in adults.

There is no RDA for manganese and therefore no specific recommendation for pregnant women. The average diet contains about 4 mg of manganese, and it is believed that an adequate daily intake is between 3 and 9 mg. These levels are easily achieved because manganese is so prevalent in many common foods, such as bananas, bran, cereal, celery, egg yolks, vegetables, liver, nuts, and pineapples.

Molybdenum

Benefits to Your Baby: **Mobilizes iron from the liver. Aids in removal of nitrogenous wastes through urea.**

Molybdenum is a trace mineral that is relatively rare, but appears in small concentrations in almost all plant and animal tissues. The mineral is a cofactor in several important enzyme systems, such as those involved in energy production, urine formation, the liberation of iron from the liver, and the oxidation of fats. Molybdenum is also required for copper metabolism.

Its role in the liberation of iron makes it an important contributor to haemoglobin production. Haemoglobin is the part of the red blood cell that carries oxygen to all other cells. However, unlike other trace minerals, there is no known set of deficiency symptoms for this mineral. There is only speculation that molybdenum can be toxic in excessive amounts, and the symptoms relate to improper copper metabolism—diarrhoea, anaemia, and depressed growth rate.

Unfortunately, there just has not been as much research with molybdenum as there has been with other minerals.

The RDA for molybdenum is 150-500 mcg for pregnant women. The mineral is found in meats, grains, legumes, milk, and green, leafy vetetables. Multivitamin-multimineral tablets may contain small amounts of molybdenum, but it is not a common addition to supplements. Therefore, eating a balanced diet should provide the required amounts of this mineral.

Phosphorus

Benefits to Your Baby: Essential to muscular and heart function. Helps build bones and teeth. Prevents blood clots by removing fatty acids from system.

Phosphorus is one of the most abundant minerals in the body. It is so readily available to every cell that there is more of a chance of an overdose of phosphorus than of a deficiency. However, phosphorus toxicity rarely causes major health problems, except that the body becomes unable to use calcium efficiently. This is because of the close relationship between calcium and phosphorus.

The body maintains a specific ratio of calcium to phosphorus in the bones. This ratio is one part calcium to one part phosphorus, and it must be the same at all times for the body to use these minerals effectively. If the ratio were to change; it should change in favour of more calcium than phosophorus. The body can easily manage a 2.5:1 calcium to phosphorus. Coincidentally, the 2.5:1 ratio is virtually identical to the ratio of these minerals in breast milk, which is usually the infant's only source of nourishment early in life.

It is phosphorus and calcium that gives bones and teeth their rigidity. Skeletal tissue contains about 80 percent of the body's phosphorus, with the rest distributed in body fluids and soft tissues. Phosphorus is involved in all chemical reactions in the body. These include the metabolism of carbohydrates, fats, and proteins for the growth, maintenance, and repair of cells, and for energy production. Phosphorus is needed for proper muscular contraction, including that of the heart. The mineral also helps the heart by breaking up and transporting fatty acids out of the body, thereby preventing blood clots.

Phosphorus is necessary for the digestion and absorption of niacin and riboflavin, two of the B complex vitamins. The mineral is also involved in cell division and reproduction, and the transfer of genetic traits from parents to children. Other functions of phosphorus include efficient nervous system transmission, the prevention of an acid or alkaline build-up in the blood, the promotion of the secretion of glandular hormones, and proper kidney function.

Phosphorus is easily absorbed by the intestines, so a deficiency is rare. In fact, more than three-quarters of the phosphorus we receive from food is absorbed by the body. This is in contrast to calcium, which is poorly absorbed. The difference in absorption rates makes it all the more imperative to maintain a proper calcium-phosphorus balance. One way the body accomplishes this is to excrete excess phosphorus in the urine. You can help keep this balance by eating foods that are rich in calcium and vitamin D.

You need phosphorus for all of your systems to function effectively, and your baby needs the mineral to promote cell and bone growth and development, muscular and heart function, and proper nervous system activity. The RDA of phosphorus for pregnant women is the same as that of calcium, which is 1,200-1,600 mg. Foods that are rich in phosphorus include eggs, fish, grains, meats, poultry, cheese, dairy products, nuts, and legumes. Phosphorus is also usually found in multimineral supplements and in individual symptoms of phosphorus are rare, they can occur. Some deficiency symptoms are loss of appetite, fatigue, possible arthritic conditions, breathing difficulties, nervous disorders, weight problems, stunted growth in children due to improper skeletal development, increased susceptibility to stress, and tooth and gum disorders. Toxicity symptoms, as mentioned earlier, would involve an improper skeletal development, increased susceptibility to stress, and tooth and gum disorders. Toxicity symptoms, as mentioned earlier, would also involve an improper utilization of calcium. Supplementation of these minerals is common, even though they are readily available in our food supply. Never supplement without a doctor's supervision. The roles of phosphorus, and calcium for that matter, are too varied and too important to arbitrarily decide how much is right for you and your baby.

Potassium

Benefits to Your Baby: Works with sodium to regulate fluid balance. Helps prevent colic and constipation. Regulates muscle function and heartbeat.

Potassium is an essential mineral that is one of the most abundant in the body. In fact, potassium makes up five percent of the total mineral content of the body. The main function of potassium is to work in conjunction with sodium to regulate the body's fluid balance. Other functions include aiding normal growth, stimulating nerve impulses for muscle contractions (including the heart's), and maintaining the alkalinity of the body. This mineral is also involved in the conversion of glucose to glycogen for storage in the liver, assisting in metabolism, enzyme reactions, and the removal of poisonous wastes from the kidney.

Potassium is best known as a counterbalance to sodium in normal heart functioning and blood pressure regulation. It has always been thought that too much sodium resulted in high blood pressure. That may be true for some people, but recent research has shown that too little potassium, even in the presence of normal sodium levels, can also result in high blood pressure. It is important to maintain appropriate intake of both sodium and potassium to ensure that both minerals function optimally.

There is no established RDA for potassium, but between 1.9 and 5.8 grams is considered safe and adequate. The best gauge is for potassium intake always to equal sodium intake. When sodium intake exceeds potassium intake, there is a tendency for potassium to be excreted in the urine. This leads to potassium deficiencies. Some of the symptoms are allergic reactions, colic in infants, constipation, diabetes, high blood pressure, heart disease, insomnia, nervous disorders, muscular disorders, slow and irregular heartbeat, and general weakness due to an inefficient metabolism. Conversely, ingestion of too much potassium can lead to anxiety, low blood pressure, cardia arrhythmias, weakness, confusion, and a possible loss of feeling in the extremeties.

Foods rich in potassium are dates, figs, peaches, tomato juice, blackstrap molasses, raisins, seafood, bananas, potatoes, wheat germ, nuts, orange juice, and sunflower seeds. The problem is that many people eat processed foods, and processing tends to remove potassium while adding sodium. This can obviously create a harmful imbalance within the body. The solution is to eat as many natural foods as possible and to take potassium supplements if necessary. However, supplementation must be under the guidance of your doctor because the correct dosage of potassium is crucial. Overdoses in certain instances may prove as dangerous as a drug overdose.

Selenium

Benefits to Your Baby: Protects cells against oxidation. Aids heart function. Helps synthesize protein in both liver and red blood cells. May protect against cancer. May protect against cot death. Protects against pollution.

Selenium is an essential trace mineral that was once considered poisonous for human consumption. This was more due to a lack of understanding of the function of this mineral than to the results of scientific research. Selenium assists vitamin

E in its metabolic role in normal physiological growth and fertility. Selenium, like vitamin E, is an antioxidant and it preserves the life of cells by delaying the time it takes for them to be burned for energy. This function may allow the mineral to play an important role in the prevention of heart disease and cancer. Selenium is necessary for the production of prostaglandin, which is a substance that affects blood pressure by keeping the arteries free from plaque (fat deposits that lead to atherosclerosis).

Some of the other functions of selenium include supplying oxygen to all cells, including muscle cells and the heart; maintenance of the health of red blood cells; DNA and RNA synthesis; cellular respiration; energy production and transfer; production of sperm cells; foetal development (may prevent cot death); health of the skin, hair, and immune system. Selenium's role as an antioxidant has caused it to be classified as an anti-aging mineral. This may or may not be true, but selenium is of great importance to a person's overall health and well-being.

There is always a possibility of selenium deficiencies because the selenium content of food depends upon the mineral content of the soil or additions to animal feed. Furthermore, selenium is easily lost in foods by processing, cooking, or simply heating. Deficiency symptoms include increased susceptibility to heart disease and possibly cancer, muscular aches and pains, rapid aging of the skin and other body systems, infertility in males, infertility in females by foetal death and resorbtion, weaknesses in cell walls leading to increased susceptibility to disease, an increase in vitamin E metabolism that causes an even greater need for the vitamin, and oxidation of the lungs and eyes in infants.

Added to selenium's other benefits that it seems to offer a protective effect against pollution by certain toxic metals, including mercury, cadmium, silver, thallium, and lead. The RDA for selenium for pregnant women is 50-200 mcg, and this can be achieved by eating fish, brewer's yeast, whole grains, organ meats, cereals, and nuts. However, remember that cooking and processing remove selenium from foods. Therefore, it may be necessary to supplement your diet with selenium, but only under the supervision of your doctor.

Silicon

Benefits to Your Baby: May strengthen bones and enhance their development. May aid in a more rapid recovery after childbirth.

Silicon is mentioned briefly here because it is such an abundant mineral that is present in the baby's connective tissue. It is possible that this mineral combines with calcium to strengthen bones and enhance their development, which would be a preventative factor in osteoporosis. Silicon also plays a role in preventing aging, speeding up the wound-healing process, maintaining proper growth and development, and possibly preventing heart disease. It performs this last function by being present in artery walls, thereby reducing the chances of atherosclerosis. When hardening of the arteries does occur, silicon levels are found to be very low.

There is no RDA for silicon. However, the mineral is so abundant in fibre-rich foods and hard drinking water that it is difficult to have a silicon deficiency. The mineral is also found in supplemental tablets. No toxic effects of silicon have been reported, but any supplementation should be done with care and professional guidance.

Sodium

Benefits to Your Baby: Works with potassium to regulate fluid balance within cells and muscle contraction.

Sodium is an essential mineral that can be both beneficial and harmful, almost at the same time. We know the relationship between high sodium intake and high blood pressure, and the negative health consequences. We also know that the prime function of sodium is to regulate the fluid and nutrient balance within cells. Sodium works with potassium to equalize the acid-alkaline balance in the body, to regulate water balance, to control nervous system transmission, and to regulate muscular contraction and expansion.

Sodium serves other important functions related to the fluids in the body. It helps keep other blood minerals soluble, so they will not build up as deposits in blood vessels. Sodium also combines with chlorine to keep blood and lymph cells healthy, remove carbon dioxide from the body, and assist in digestion through the production of hydrochloric acid in the stomach. Finally, sodium, in the form of salt, will not cause toxemia of pregnancy, a condition whose symptoms can cause blurred vision, a rise in blood pressure, a presence of abnormal substances in the urine, headaches and sudden weight gain.

It is difficult to have a sodium deficiency because almost all foods contain some sodium, and food processing adds sodium. If a deficiency were to occur, some of the symptoms would be intestinal gas, appetite loss, dehydration, fever, muscle shrinkage, weight loss, vomiting, and improper carbohydrate metabolism. The other side of the fence is excessive sodium intake. This occurs by eating too many processed foods and adding too much salt to food. Toxic symptoms include high blood pressure, potassium loss, abnormal fluid retention, dizziness, and swelling.

There is no RDA for sodium, but most people ingest about 3–7 grams a day. Most of this comes in the form of salt, and it is far in excess of what is actually needed. You should take it about one gram of salt for every 2 pints of water consumed. Be aware that sodium must be part of your diet because it is essential for the proper functioning of your body and your baby's body. Sodium prevents muscle cramps, heat cramps, and heat stroke, and it helps preserve nerve strength. Sodium is also stored in the bones along with calcium, and it helps calcium maintain the integrity of the skeletal system.

Sulphur

Benefits to Your Baby: Necessary for tissue respiration, energy production and the secretion of bile. Aids in the production of haemoglobin. Is a component of protein and assists in all its functions.

Sulphur is stored in every cell of the body and it makes up about .25 percent of total body weight. The mineral plays several important roles in maintaining health. It is a component of protein and assists in all of its functions. Sulphur also works with thiamine, pantothenic acid, biotin, and lipoic acid to improve metabolism and nerve health. It is necessary for tissue respiration, energy production, the secretion of bile from the liver, and the health of the hair, skin, and nails. Finally, sulphur aids in the production of haemoglobin.

There is no RDA for sulphur because it is assumed that the body's requirements are met when protein intake is at the required level. Thus, deficiency symptoms are almost nonexistent, but if they were to occur, the most obvious signs would be skin disorders. In fact, ointments containing sulphur are used to treat skin disorders such as eczema, psoriasis, and dermatitis. The best food source of sulphur is eggs, with other goods sources being bran, cheese, clams, nuts, fish, and wheat-germ.

Zinc

Benefits to Your Baby: Important component in growth of skeletal system and nervous system. Component of insulin. Speeds the healing process and assists in digestion. Aids in development of reproductive organs, connective tissue, and protects the baby's cells.

Zinc is fast becoming known as the 'wonder mineral.' It is involved in at least forty different enzyme systems, covering every major physiological function of the body. Zinc is responsible for helping the body absorb the B complex vitamins, plus it assists in digestion, metabolism, and tissue respiration. Zinc is a component of insulin and part of the enzyme that breaks down alcohol in the body. The mineral plays a major role in the synthesis of DNA, RNA, and protein. Zinc is required for cell growth, the formation of connective tissue, proper development of the reproductive organs, general growth functions, protection of cells (perhaps through an antioxidant effect), and the healing of burns and wounds. In fact, zinc compounds in local applications have been used to speed up the healing process.

When there is not enough zinc in the system, there is delayed healing of wounds and growth processes are slowed. Deformities occur in infants whose mothers are deficient in zinc. There is impaired development of the neuromuscular and skeletal systems, delayed sexual maturity, loss of hair, deformed nails, acne and skin lesions, increased susceptibility to fatigue and stress, infertility, atrophy of the thymus gland, and reduced absorption of nutrients. The possibility exists that a zinc deficiency can lead to an increased risk of atherosclerosis because the zinc may eliminate the cholesterol deposits that cause this disease, a predisposition to cancer, and a decrease in mental alertness. The baby whose mother is zinc deficient will probably be born with nervous system and skeletal malformations.

There are some warning signs of a zinc deficiency. These include stretch marks on the skin, white spots on the fingernails, brittle nails and hair, loss of hair pigment, irregular menstrual cycles, and painful joints (a possible precursor to arthritis, which seems to be alleviated by zinc intake). The damage that is done by prolonging a zinc deficiency can be irreparable. This is especially true for a pregnant woman, since her developing foetus relies so heavily on an adequate zinc supply for proper growth and development.

The RDA for zinc is 15 mg for nonpregnant women and 20–25 mg for pregnant women. There are some instances in which zinc requirements for a pregnant woman may be higher, but that must be determined by a doctor. Children also have RDAs for this mineral because it is so vital to everyone's overall health. Infants up to five months old need 3 mg of zinc a day, those who are five months to one year require 5 mg, and children up to ten years old should have 10 mg a day. The best sources of zinc are brewer's yeast, liver, seafood, soya beans, spinach, mushrooms, and sunflower seeds. Unfortunately, most diets are marginally deficient in zinc. Therefore, zinc supplementation is recommended under a doctor's supervision. This is suggested even though there is no known toxicity for zinc.

One final word should be mentioned regarding zinc. It is true this mineral performs many vital functions. However, that does not mean zinc is a 'wonder mineral.' It is an essential mineral that works in conjunction with other nutrients to give you your best chance for achieving optimal health.

Other Minerals

There are several other minerals, but we won't talk about them here. This is because either not much is known about them or they do not offer the benefits to you and your baby that the minerals already mentioned provide. Some of these other minerals are aluminum, beryllium, bismuth, cadmium, cobalt, lead, mercury, nickel, strontium, tin, and vanadium. These minerals do serve functions, but they are not considered to be as vital to optimal health during pregnancy as the minerals described above.

3

Exercise and Pregnancy

Exercise during pregnancy is especially important. You are experiencing considerable weight gain and neuromuscular and structural changes. Exercise helps you deal with those changes more comfortably. This is done through a basic exercise programme that emphasizes muscle strengthening and toning, some stretching, and cardiovascular conditioning. Participation in a prenatal exercise programme does not guarantee an easy labour or a faster postpartum recovery. However, exercise during pregnancy may provide you with more stamina to endure labour and delivery, better circulation, better posture and respiration, greater body awareness, a higher energy level, and a quicker and easier return to prepregnant size and strength levels.

The goals of an exercise programme for pregnant women appear to be straightforward and simple. The programme must be designed to increase muscle strength and endurance, specifically those muscles that are most affected by pregnancy, labour, and delivery. This includes the abdominals, the low back muscles, and those of the pelvic floor. On the other hand, the pregnancy exercise programme must be designed to enable you to carry out your activities in comfort. This is the most difficult aspect of the programme because it depends on many factors. These include the type of activities you are involved in, your present condition and medical history, and your response to exercise and pregnancy based on that history. What type of exercise programme will bring about the desired results while avoiding the potential dangers of physical exercise during pregnancy—including the possibility of dehydration, hyperthermia, hypoxia, energy drain, and injury? Also, are trained personnel available to alter the exercise programme to meet the progressive physical demands of pregnancy?

The cardiovascular portion of the exercise program should maintain your prepregnant aerobic condition, depending on the level of that condition. There is no need to improve fitness levels. Rather, it is more important to maintain fitness levels. Finally, the programme must be geared to the individual. Women enter pregnancy in different physical condition. Some were active and fit prior to becoming pregnant, while others were only moderately active, and still others were sedentary. The key is to have each woman know her fitness levels and train within her capabilities.

Pregnancy Exercise Concerns

There are many concerns related to exercise during pregnancy, concerns voiced by pregnant women and their doctors. Much research has been done to support or refute these concerns because exercise is such an important part of everyone's life. Many pregnant women who were active before they became pregnant continue their activities, sometimes despite their doctor's recommendations. If your doctor's request is made because of a medical condition or complication, then continuing exercise is not a wise move on your part. If the request is made because of incomplete knowledge related to exercise and pregnancy, then you have to listen to your body and continue doing what makes you feel good.

The primary concern people have about exercise during pregnancy is the effect all that activity will have on the developing foetus. The premise is that the mother can take care of herself, but no one seems to know how the foetus will be affected. Modern medical technology has allowed us to study the effects of maternal exercise on the foetus, and we know that certain environmental changes do occur. Maternal levels of catecholamines, the stress hormones, increase, as do the levels of lactic acid. Serum glucose levels decrease, and perhaps most importantly, uterine blood flow decreases. These changes may not affect the mother greatly, but the manner in which they influence foetal development can be paramount. The increased catecholamines tend to alter the foetal heart rate, first speeding it up and then, as more blood and oxygen are diverted to the mother's working muscles, slowing it down. The increased lactic acid makes it harder for the mother's muscles to work properly, the decreased glucose levels lead to a drop in energy for both mother and baby, and the decreased uterine blood flow may lead to a diminished supply to the foetus.

These concerns may appear to be dramatic but they are not really dangerous to the foetus. The changes in foetal heart rate are only temporary during each exercise period and do not seem to have a detrimental effect on birth outcome. The same is true for the diminished or diverted uterine blood supply. The mother's body tends to compensate for this by increasing the oxygen concentration and iron concentration of each unit of blood that it sends to the foetus during exercise. Therefore, while the total volume of blood may be decreased, the amount of nourishment remains basically the same.

Finally, some active pregnant women who continue exercising up to the point of labour with weight-bearing exercises such as jogging tend to give birth to slightly lower birth-weight babies. This lower weight does not usually affect the health and well-being of the infant. Rather, it probably results because more of the mother's calories are used for energy during exercise and less are distributed to the foetus. Also, exercise speeds up the metabolism, and the mother who exercises probably burns more calories at rest than her sedentary or less active counterpart. However, if you are concerned about the lower birthweight, then you should emphasize non-weight-bearing exercises such as cycling, swimming, and strength training. This will allow you to continue to be active and to maintain your muscular and cardiovascular fitness, and your baby will be delivered at the same birthweight as if you had not been exercising at all.

One important recommendation must be made at this point. The concerns over the relationship between exercise and pregnancy are valid if they are pertinent to your specific condition. However, there is one benefit of exercise that may far outweigh any of the concerns. If exercise makes you feel better about yourself, even without any other physiological changes or benefits, then a safe pregnancy exercise programme is worthwhile and even advisable.

Safe Exercise Guidelines

It is only recently that there has been a boom in exercise classes and programmes for pregnant women. This seems to be a consequence of the fact that these women were active before pregnancy and simply wanted to continue with their physical fitness programme. Some of the exercise classes that were organized followed the typical exercise prescription for normal healthy adults: a minimum of three times a week for 15 to 60 minutes each session with the heart rate in its target training zone. (Your target heart rate can be found by subtracting your age from 220 and multiplying the number by .7 to .85) (220 − age x .7 to .85). This general prescription is good by healthy, asymptomatic individuals, but people began to realize that pregnant women are a special group. Pregnancy exercise programmes began to be designed based on theoretical, practical, scientific, and anecdotal evidence. These more sophisticated programs became popular, so much so that the medical community started to take notice. Doctors then decided to become involved in the development of guidelines for such exercise.

The American College of Sports Medicine, perhaps the

best-known and most respected fitness association in the world, developed guidelines under which people could enter into an exercise programme. Basically, anyone who is under 45 years of age, with no evidence or history of cardiovascular disease and no primary or secondary risk factors for coronary artery disease, and has had a medical evaluation within the last year is eligible to participate in an exercise programme without further medical clearance. People at or above age 45 or who have one or more risk factors should first be evaluated by a doctor and an exercise physiologist to determine their capabilities for physical activity. The college also specified an extensive list of contraindications (not to be done) and relative contraindications (only to be done under certain conditions) to exercise. Any person possessing a contraindication would be forbidden to exercise, except perhaps under close medical supervision. The problem with all these guidelines and specifications is that no mention is made of pregnancy.

Several of the original guidelines and contraindications can be adapted for pregnancy. Common sense dictates that if you have any of the following risk factors or contraindications you should not begin an exercise programme without a comprehensive medical evaluation. These risk factors include any form of heart disease, high blood pressure, pulmonary disease, premature labour potential, uterine bleeding, anaemia, diabetes (not gestational), breech presentation during the last 3 months, and suspected foetal distress. Any additional contraindications must be left up to your doctor. Finally, you should realize that you are susceptible to the same types of musculoskeletal injuries as anyone else, plus you have the possibility of inducing premature labour towards the end of the last 3 months.

It was probably these considerations that led the American College of Obstetricians and Gynaecologists to develop and introduce guidelines for exercise during pregnancy. These guidelines have been criticized, primarily because they are general and do not account for possible individual differences. Also, several of them are not based on scientific fact, and there are so many constraints that an exercise programme that adheres to these guidelines to the letter would probably not tax a physically fit woman who has become pregnant. These complaints notwithstanding, the guidelines have been approved by the college and they at least present a starting point for a pregnancy exercise programme. They are presented here only for your information and not as an endorsement of any or all of them. That determination is up to you and your doctor.

Guidelines for Exercise During Pregnancy and Postpartum

- Regular exercise (at least three times a week) is preferable to intermittent activity. Competitive activities should be discouraged.
- Vigorous exercise should not be performed in hot, humid weather or during an illness when a fever is present.
- Ballistic movements (jerky, bouncy motions) should be avoided. Exercises should be done on a wooden floor or a tightly carpeted surface to reduce shock and provide sure footing.
- Deep flexion or extension of joints should be avoided because of connective tissue laxity. Activities that require jumping, jarring motions, or rapid changes in direction should be avoided because of joint instability.
- Vigorous exercises should be preceded by a five-minute period of muscle warm-up. This can be accomplished by slow walking or stationary cycling with low resistance.
- Vigorous exercise should be followed by a period of gradually declining activity that includes gentle stationary stretching. Because connective tissue laxity increases the risk of joint injury, stretches should not be taken to the point of maximum resistance.
- Heart rate should be measured at times of peak activity. Target heart rates and limits established in consultation with the physician should not be exceeded.

- Care should be taken to rise gradually from the floor to avoid orthostatic hypotension (dizziness due to a change in posture). Some form of activity involving the legs should be continued for a brief period.
- Liquids should be taken liberally before and after exercise to prevent dehydration. If necessary, activity should be interrupted to replenish fluids.
- Women who have led sedentary lifestyles should begin with physical activity of very low intensity and advance activity levels very gradually.
- Activity should be stopped and the physician consulted if any unusual symptoms appear.

Pregnancy Only

- Maternal heart rate should not exceed 140 beats per minute.
- Strenuous activities should not exceed 15 minutes in duration.
- No exercise should be performed in the supine position (lying on the back) after the fourth month of gestation (pregnancy).
- Exercises that employ the Valsalva manoeuvre (exhaling while keeping your mouth closed and holding your breath) should be avoided.
- Calorie intake should be adequate to meet not only the extra energy needs of pregnancy but also of the exercise performed.
- Maternal core temperatures should not exceed 38 degrees Centigrade (100.4 degrees Farenheit).

It is true that the guidelines are conservative, but this may be a positive rather than a negative factor. Since exercise during pregnancy is still a relatively new field, it is best to err on the side of conservatism. Of course, only you and your doctor can determine your actual physical limitations during exercise. Therefore, if you wish to begin an exercise programme, research it, see if it will meet your needs, determine if it is safe by possibly using the guidelines above as a checklist, and then enter the program with your doctor's approval. One other factor may be helpful in selecting a programme, and this is true for pregnant as well as nonpregnant women. There is a table in Appendix C that lists 25 exercises to avoid and what parts of the body can be injured if these exercises are performed. Stay away from any exercise programme that includes several or all of these exercises.

Exercise Sessions

All exercise sessions should consist of a warm-up, a muscle conditioning period, an aerobic or cardiovascular conditioning period, and a cool-down. This is true whether you are participating in an exercise or aerobics class or simply working out on your own. Putting these components into an exercise session in their proper sequence will ensure a safe and effective workout.

The warm-up is designed to loosen up the major muscle groups that will be used during the exercise session. Warm-ups should consist of low-intensity, rhythmic range-of-motion activities that mimic the more strenuous exercises you will perform during the conditioning session. Stretching should be done only toward the end of the warm-up, when the core temperature of the muscles has been raised sufficiently to make them more supple and pliable. If you stretch before warming up, you can easily tear a cold muscle. The best analogy is trying to stretch a rubber band that has been sitting in your freezer; it snaps quickly and easily.

The calisthenic conditioning period or weight/strength training period should consist of all the muscle-building exercises that are normally part of your workout schedule. The best advice here is to work from the larger muscle groups to the smaller ones. Also, never go for the 'burn,' as that can increase susceptibility to injuries more than it can build up muscle strength. This period is followed by cardiovascular conditioning, where the progression is from moderate intensity exercises to more vigorous ones. The important point here is to stay within your training heart-rate range, which is usually defined as 220 minus your age multiplied by 70 and 85 percent. If you are following the guidelines here, your heart rate should never exceed 140 beats a minute, regardless of the appropriate training zone.

The cool-down is the last part of the exercise session and it should be a mirror image of the warm-up. Low-intensity, rhythmic range-of-motion exercises should be performed to allow the heat rate to drop toward resting levels. These types of activities also prevent blood from pooling in the extremities. Any stretching that is to be done during the cool-down should be done from a standing position, and the head should never be below the heart. This is especially important for pregnant women.

These components of an exercise session will produce desired fitness results for both pregnant and nonpregnant women. The effectiveness of any exercise programme is directly related to the individual exercise prescription, which is the number of times an exercise is performed each week (frequency), how hard you must work during the exercise session (intensity), and how long the exercise session lasts (time or duration). Frequency, intensity, and time (FIT) are the most important determinants of a successful exercise programme. Women must also choose their activity carefully. It must be one they prefer and enjoy. Therefore, once you determined your exercise prescription and programme with the advice of your doctor, it is up to you to identify those activities you enjoy the most. In that way, you will assure yourself of all the benefits that exercise during pregnancy can bring.

Benefits of Exercise

Exercise has been called the panacea of life. There are claims that exercise can prevent heart disease and cancer, extend life, cure illness, and improve work productivity. Some of these claims are true at certain times for specific people, but not everyone will receive these types of benefits just because they exercise. However, there are more than 100 substantiated exercise benefits for both pregnant and nonpregnant women. Some of the more important ones are improved fitness levels or at least maintenance of prepregnant fitness levels, greater muscular endurance and strength so that labour and delivery can be better tolerated, prevention of excessive weight gain during pregnancy, improved posture and decreased backache, increased self-esteem, improved ability to manage stress, quicker recovery from postpartum depression and physical status, improved digestion and circulation leading to a decrease in nausea and varicose veins, and more restful sleep. Remember that these are only some of the benefits that exercise can offer you. There certainly are many more, since pregnant women will also receive most of the benefits of their nonpregnant counterparts. The key for you is to realize that exercise can help your pregnancy, but it must be done in moderation and preferably under a doctor's care.

Doctors who are aware of the benefits of exercise to pregnancy will emphasize a muscle strengthening programme over a cardiovascular conditioning programme. They are not ignoring the importance of cardiovascular exercises. Rather, they realize that aerobic conditioning during pregnancy should be more of a maintenance programme one than to improve endurance. Pregnant women should emphasize muscle strengthening and muscular endurance exercises. This is to minimize the risk of joint and ligament injuries, to correct and improve posture, to avoid muscle strain, and to condition the muscles that are responsible for carrying the baby, labour, and delivery. The muscles that are most important during pregnancy include those of the pelvic floor, the abdominals, and the lower back. All pregnancy exercise programs should emphasize these areas, with a secondary emphasis on strengthening the other muscle groups.

There are many programmes today that claim to follow

all the guidelines mentioned above and focus on the muscle groups that are important. Some of these are merely exercise classes for pregnant women, with no theoretical or scientific background. Others are medically oriented and supervised.

Conclusions

Exercise during pregnancy is a relatively new aspect of physical fitness training. Most women are active in their prepregnant state and wish to remain so throughout their pregnancy. They are aware of the obvious physical and psychological benefits of exercise during pregnancy, such as not gaining too much weight, returning to a prepregnant figure more rapidly, feeling better about themselves, and actually looking better throughout the pregnancy. These women, and others who were sedentary or moderately active before becoming pregnant, are now also realizing the importance of participating in physical conditioning programs so that they can enjoy a safer pregnancy. Proper exercises during pregnancy will maintain cardiovascular fitness while strengthening those muscle groups that are primarily used to carry the foetus and to go through labour and delivery. There is both scientific and anecdotal evidence that women who exercise during pregnancy experience less intense pain and have a shorter labour and delivery period.

Pregnant women who wish to achieve these exercise benefits must first receive their doctor's permission to exercise, then they must research all the available programmes. A sound programme is one that is based on medical and scientific research, is staffed by trained professionals, does not offer exercises that are potentially harmful, and that follows some type of accepted guidelines for exercise during pregnancy, such as those proposed by the American College of Obstetricians and Gynecologists. Once a programme is selected on the basis of these criteria, pregnant women should follow the suggestions below to receive the greatest benefit from their participation:

1 Perform exercises slowly and through the full range of motion so that the joints are protected from strain.
2 Monitor the intensity of the exercise session carefully. Never overexert yourself, and stop exercising if you feel dizzy, faint, breathless, or light-headed.
3 Always breathe properly during exercise. Never hold your breath.
4 Avoid activities that require rapid changes of direction of shifts in balance.
5 Avoid exercises that increase swayback or place an excess strain on the back.
6 Keep exercises simple, as coordination and balance are changing. Always maintain proper alignment and posture, and switch positions often to prevent muscles from becoming fatigued.
7 Decrease weight-bearing exercises as pregnancy progresses and concentrate on non-weight-bearing exercises such as cycling, swimming, stretching, or weight training with machines.
8 Avoid risky activities and sports in which the chance of injury is increased.
9 Wear supportive shoes and a supportive bra during exercise to make the routines more comfortable and to help maintain proper posture.
10 Drink plenty of fluids before, during, and after exercise and make sure you are eating enough to compensate for the extra energy expenditure.

These are some basic suggestions for pregnant women to follow while participating in an exercise programme. There is a more extensive list in Appendix C that applies to both pregnant and nonpregnant women. Proper and safe exercise will result in a more enjoyable pregnancy, a shorter labour and delivery, and a faster return to prepregnant fitness.

4

Summary

The benefits of exercise during pregnancy are many, and the contributions of exercise to a healthier lifestyle have filled many volumes. However, we must not forget that the pregnant woman is eating for two, and that she must provide herself and her unborn baby with the proper nourishment. This means she must eat right, eat light, eat often from the basic food groups, and take her vitamins and minerals daily. The beneficial effects of taking vitamins and minerals, either through food ingestion or supplementation, have been demonstrated throughout this book. It is a well-known fact that pregnancy places additional and unusual demands upon the mother-to-be that cannot be met by simply eating a 'balanced diet' that provides the basic RDAs. This is obvious because the RDAs for pregnant women are greater for almost all the vitamins and minerals than those recommended for their nonpregnant counterparts. Therefore, unless you can be certain you are getting all the necessary vitamins and minerals from the foods you eat, you will have to supplement your diet. Remember, though, never supplement without the guidance of a doctor. It is only through medical supervision and appropriate vitamin and mineral supplementation that you can be assured of a healthy pregnancy.

5

Questions and Answers

Can I take vitamins and minerals in place of meals?
Vitamins and minerals are food supplements, not meal replacements. They are never to be taken instead of a meal. Vitamins and minerals have no calorific value. Only food contains calories, and calories are needed for energy by both you and your baby. The vitamins and minerals help you metabolize the food and turn the calories into usable energy. Therefore, supplements should be taken only in conjunction with food, and preferably after a meal.

Is there a difference between natural and synthetic vitamins and which ones should I take during my pregnancy?
There is absolutely no difference between natural and synthetic vitamins. Vitamins are chemical compounds and they are classified as a particular vitamin based on their chemical structure. How the chemical compound came to be is unimportant. You use the vitamin the same way regardless of its origin. The only concern you should have regarding natural versus synthetic vitamins is that natural vitamins cost significantly more.

Must I take vitamins and mineral supplements if I eat a well-balanced diet throughout my pregnancy?
This is a point of controversy among nutritionists, doctors, and other professionals. There are those who suggest that a well-balanced diet will provide all the nutrients you need

in accordance with the RDAs. Others believe that the processing and cooking of foods destroys important nutrients, and that the RDAs can't be met because of this. Still others claim that the RDAs are not enough for normal, daily functioning, let alone special situations such as pregnancy. These latter groups support the use of vitamin and mineral supplements because they can cite research that shows there is maternal malnutrition in highly developed countries where 'well-balanced diets' are supposed to be easily accessible.

Perhaps the most important thing is to realize that you are an individual who will respond differently to pregnancy than anyone else. This is especially true with regard to nutritional needs. People digest food and absorb its nutrients at different rates and in different manners. Also, each foetus nourishes itself in a unique way. Some draw more heavily from the mother than others. Hence, vitamin and mineral supplements should be taken during pregnancy to ensure adequate nutrient intake for both you and your baby. Even if the supplements are not providing any noticeable physiological benefits, they may provide you with psychological benefits. You may feel better and believe the supplements are working. Even if it is only a placebo effect—but it is probably much more than that on all levels—it must be remembered that a healthy mind will create a healthy body for a healthy pregnancy.

Since vitamin and mineral supplements are beneficial, wouldn't it be better to take them in larger doses?
The old adage, 'If some is good, more is better,' does not hold true here. Megadoses of vitamins, which means taking more than ten times the RDA, are unhealthy for pregnant women. Vitamin toxicity can occur in much the same way drug toxicity occurs. When taking vitamin and mineral supplements, take only what is recommended by your doctor.

Are the supplements I take during pregnancy affecting only me or will my baby benefit also?
Both you and your baby benefit from your taking supplements. Everything you eat during your pregnancy is passed

on to the baby. In fact, when appropriate amounts of food, vitamins, and minerals are ingested, the foetus feeds from these rather than from your stored supplies.

Will exercise during pregnancy increase my need for certain vitamins and minerals?
Exercise will probably not cause an increased requirement for vitamins and minerals. What exercise will do is increase your ability to absorb and utilize nutrients. This is due to improved oxygen transport and circulation in your body. The ultimate beneficiary is your baby, which receives its nourishment from a healthy mother.

Should I keep taking supplements after I give birth?
Yes, especially if you are breast-feeding. Lactating women still have higher nutritional requirements than non-pregnant women. Also, you are still the only source of nourishment for your newborn baby. Even if you are not breast-feeding, you should maintain your supplementation. Pregnancy, labour, and delivery make exhausting demands on your system; it will take months to fully recover. Continuing your supplementation during the recovery period will help you regain full health more quickly.

Does my baby need vitamin and mineral supplements as a newborn?
Yes. Most paediatricians prescribe liquid vitamin and mineral formulas for infants. This is regardless of whether the infant is breast-fed or formula-fed. Additionally, the baby's growth rate is more rapid during the first year of life than at any other time. This rapid development requires high-quality nutrition. Supplements, given under a doctor's care, will ensure that your baby receives the appropriate vitamins and minerals in the proper doses for his or her growth.

Are vitamins and mineral supplements necessary before pregnancy?
It is a well-proven fact that a mother's prepregnant nutritional status will have a significant effect on the health of the foetus. The typical diet is not as well-balanced as everyone would like to believe. Therefore, you should try to eat properly, but

you should also take supplements to provide the nutrients that may be lacking in your diet.

Will vitamins help me have a 'super baby'?
The answer is an emphatic no. Supplementation cannot create or guarantee a 'super baby.' Only genetics, hard work, and a little bit of luck can do that. It is more important to have a healthy baby than a 'super baby.'

What is the best vitamin and mineral supplement to take during pregnancy?
There is no single best brand of supplement. You should be aware of your increased need for iron, folacin, vitamin C, calcium, phosphorus, magnesium, zinc, and vitamin B complex to name some of the nutrients that are especially required for a healthy pregnancy. The supplement you take should fulfill your individual needs. It is wise to discuss these needs with your doctor so that the proper supplements and their dosages can be prescribed. Then it is up to you to comply with the prescription and take the supplements when they are supposed to be taken.

Should I take a multivitamin tablet and a multimineral tablet or a combination, or should I take each vitamin and mineral in single tablet form?
It is best to take a combination multivitamin and multimineral tablet because vitamins and minerals work in conjunction. You may take a specific vitamin or mineral as a single tablet if your doctor feels that the additional supplementation is necessary. It is costly, time-consuming, and potentially unhealthy to take all your vitamins and minerals in single-tablet form. Remember to choose the multiple tablet that best suits your needs and your baby's needs.

Appendix A: Vitamin and Mineral Chart

Vitamin/Mineral	Daily Dosage	Sources	Deficiency Symptoms	Benefits
A Fat-Soluble	RDA: 5,000 IU SR: 10,000–25,000 IU Toxicity: 50,000 IU P&L: 5,000–8,000 IU	Green and yellow fruits and vegetables, milk, milk products, fish liver oil, apricots (dried), beef liver, spinach, raw carrots	Allergies, appetite loss, asthma, bronchitis, colds, fatigue, heart disease, hepatitis, night blindness, stress, susceptibility to infections	Aids bone and tissue growth and cell development, maintains health of skin and mucous membranes for mother and baby throughout pregnancy
B Complex	RDA: see B vitamins SR: see B vitamins Toxicity: not known P&L: 1.5–1.6 mg	Brewer's yeast, liver, whole grains	Anaemia, allergies, constipation, digestive disturbances, heart abnormalities, hypoglycaemia, insomnia overweight, stress	Enhances nervous system development and energy metabolism
B1 Thiamine Water-Soluble	RDA: 1–1.5 mg SR: 2–10 mg Toxicity: not known P&L: 1.5–1.6 mg	Blackstrap molasses, brewer's yeast, brown rice, fish, meat, nuts, organ meats, poultry, wheat germ, peanuts, sunflower seeds, Brazil nuts	Appetite loss, congestive heart failure, constipation, diabetes, digestive disturbances, fatigue, nausea, nervousness, rapid heart rate, pain and noise sensitivity, shortness of breath, stress	Determines rate at which energy is released from stored sugar

Vitamin/Mineral	Daily Dosage	Sources	Deficiency Symptoms	Benefits
B2 Riboflavin Water-Soluble	RDA: 1.3-1.7 mg SR: 2-10 mg Toxicity: not known P&L: 1.5-1.8 mg	Blackstrap molasses, nuts, organ meats, whole grains, almonds, brussel sprouts, brewer's yeast, beef liver	Diabetes, diarrhoea, indigestion, retarded growth	Aids in energy and protein metabolism.
Niacin Niacinamide (B Complex) Water-Soluble	RDA: 13-18 mg SR: 50-5,000 mg Toxicity: not known P&L: 15-20 mg	Brewer's yeast, seafood, lean meats, milk, milk products, poultry, dessicated liver, rhubarb (cooked), chicken (breast, fried), peanuts (roasted with skin)	Appetite loss, depression diarrhoea, fatigue, headaches, high blood pressure, indigestion, insomnia, leg cramps, migraine headaches, muscular weakness, nausea, nervous disorders, poor circulation, stress	Coenzyme in energy and protein metabolism.
B6 Pyridoxine Water-Soluble	RDA: 1.8-2.2 mg SR: 4-50 mg Toxicity: not known P&L: 2.5 mg	Blackstrap molasses, brewer's yeast, green leafy vegetables, meat, organ meats, wheat germ, whole grains, dessicated liver, beef liver, prunes (cooked), brown rice, peas	Anaemia, atherosclerosis, convulsions in babies, depression, gestational diabetes, hypoaglycemia, irritability, learning disabilities, mental retardation, muscular disorders, nervous disorders, nausea in pregnancy, obesity	Helps control nausea. Foetus requires B6 for growth. Also acts as a coenzyme in amino acid metabolism and protein synthesis. May prevent heart disease.

Vitamin	Dosage	Sources	Deficiency	Function
B12 Cobalimin Water-Soluble	RDA: 3 mcg SR: 5–50 mg Toxicity: not known P&L: 4 mcg	Cheese, fish, milk, milk products, organ meats, cottage cheese, liver, tuna fish (canned), eggs	**Allergies, anaemia, bronchial asthma,** fatigue, general weakness, hypoglycaemia, insomnia, nervousness, pernicious aenemia, obesity	Aids nervous system development and formation of red blood cells. Acts as a coenzyme in protein metabolism.
B15 Pangamic Acid Water-Soluble	RDA: non stated SR: not known Toxicity: not known P&L: 2.5–10 mg (estimate)	Brewer's yeast, brown rice, meat (rare), seeds (sunflower, sesame, pumpkin), whole grains, organ meats	Asthma, atherosclerosis heart disease, headaches, insomnia, nervous & glandular disorders, poor circulation, shortness of breath	May work in prevention of heart disease.
Biotin (B Complex) Water-Soluble	RDA: 150–300 mcg SR: 300–500 mg Toxicity: not known P&L: 300–500 mcg	Legumes, whole grains, organ meats, brewer's yeast, lentils, mung bean sprouts, egg yolk, beef liver, soyabeans	Depression, fatigue, insomnia, leg cramps, muscular pain, poor appetite	Prevents muscle cramping and soreness Aids muscular development and motor control. May prevent cot death.
Choline (B Complex) Water-Soluble	RDA: none stated SR: 100–1,000 mg Toxicity: not known P&L: 1,000 mg	Brewer's yeast, fish, legumes, organ meats, soyabeans, wheat germ, lecithin, beef liver, egg yolks, peanuts (roasted with skin)	Atherosclerosis, bleeding stomach ulcers, constipation, dizziness, growth problems, hardening of the arteries, headaches, high blood pressure, hypoglycaemia, impaired liver and kidney function, insomnia, intolerance to fats	Aids in circulatory system functions and memory development

Vitamin/Mineral	Daily Dosage	Sources	Deficiency Symptoms	Benefits
Folic Acid Folacin Water-Soluble	RDA: 400 mcg SR: 1,000–10,000 mcg Toxicity: not known P&L: 800 mcg	Green leafy vegetables, milk, milk products, organ meats, oysters, salmon, whole grains, brewer's yeast, dates (dried), spinach (steamed), tuna fish (canned)	Anaemia, atherosclerosis, diarrhoea, digestive disturbances, fatigue, growth problems, mental illness, stomach ulcers	Prevents anaemia along with iron. Needed for haemoglobin synthesis. Involved in synthesis of DNA and RNA. Coenzyme in amino acid synthesis.
Inositol (B Complex) Water-Soluble	RDA: none stated SR: 100–1,000 mg Toxicity: not known P&L: 1,000 mg	Blackstrap molasses, citrus fruits, brewer's yeast, meat, milk, nuts, vegetables, whole grains, lecithin, peanuts (roasted with skin)	Atherosclerosis, constipation, eye abnormalities, heart disease, obesity	Aids in development of nervous system and prevention of heart disease.
Pantothenic Acid (B Complex) Water-Soluble	RDA: 5–10 mg SR: 20–100 mg Toxicity: not known P&L: 5–10 mg	Brewer's yeast, legumes, organ meats, salmon, wheat germ, whole grains, beef liver, mushrooms (cooked), elderberries (raw), orange juice (fresh)	Allergies, colitis, diarrhoea, duodenal ulcers, digestive disorders, hypoglycaemia, intestinal disorders, kidney troubles, muscle cramps, respiratory infections, vomiting	Helps body to resist stress. Assists in production of adrenaline. May slow down biochemical aging process.

Para Amino-benzoic Acid (B Complex) Water-Soluble	RDA: none stated SR: 10–100 mg Toxicity: not known P&L: 10–30 mg (estimate)	Blackstrap molasses, brewer's yeast, liver, organ meats, wheat germ	Constipation, depression digestive disorders, fatigue, headaches, sunburn	Prevents skin wrinkling. May deter aging and cancer process.
C Ascorbic Acid Water-Soluble	RDA: 60 mg SR: 250–5,000 mg Toxicity: 5,000–15,000 mg P&L: 80 mg	Citrus fruits, cantaloupe, green peppers, broccoli (cooked), papaya (raw), strawberries	Allergies, anaemia, atherosclerosis, bleeding gums, bruises, capillary wall ruptures, colds, hypoglycaemia, heart disease, hepatitis, low infection resistance, poor digestion, obesity	Helps tissue formation and maintains integrity of immune system. 'Cement' in connective and vascular tissues. Increases iron absorption.
Bioflavonoids Water-Soluble	RDA: none stated SR: none stated Toxicity: none stated P&L: none stated	Citrus fruits, vegetables	Same as Vitamin C	Prevents excess bleeding. Enhances use of vitamin C.
D Fat-Soluble	RDA: 400 IU SR: 500–1,500 IU Toxicity: 2,500 IU P&L: 500–600 IU	Egg yolks, organ meats, bone meal, sunlight, beef liver, milk, salmon tuna (canned)	Allergies, diarrhoea, insomnia, nervousness, poor metabolism, softening bones and teeth	Aids absorption of calcium and phosphorus. Helps build strong bones and teeth

Vitamin/Mineral	Daily Dosage	Sources	Deficiency Symptoms	Benefits
E Tocopherol Fat-Soluble	RDA: 12-15 IU SR: 50-600 IU Toxicity: 4,000-40,000 IU P&L: 15 IU	Dark green vegetables, eggs, liver, organ meats, wheat germ, vegetable oils, dessicated liver, oatmeal (cooked), safflower oil, vegetable oils, peanuts (roasted with skin), tomatoes, wheat germ oil	Allergies, atherosclerosis crossed eyes, diabetes, gastrointestinal disease, heart disease (coronary thrombosis, angina pectoris, rheumatic heart disease), migraine, miscarriages, muscular wasting, obesity, thrombosis	Enhances absorption of Vitamin A. Aids tissue growth, cell wall development circulation and red blood cell integrity.
F Unsaturated fatty acids Fat-Soluble	RDA: none stated SR: 10% total calories Toxicity: not known P&L: none stated	Vegetable oils (safflower, soy, corn), wheat germ, sunflower seeds	Allergies, bronchial asthma, diarrhoea, heart disease, obesity, weight loss	Need a ratio of 2:1 unsaturated to saturated fats in the diet, to insure proper bodily functions.
K Menadione Fat-Soluble	RDA: none stated SR: 300-500 mcg Toxicity: not known P&L: none stated	Green leafy vegetables, safflower oil, blackstrap molasses, yogurt, oatmeal, beef liver	Bruises, diarrhoea, increased tendency to hamorrhage, miscarriages	Aids in blood clotting.
Calcium	RDA: 800-1,200 mg SR: 1,000-1,400 mg Toxicity: not known P&L: 1,200-1,600 mg	Milk, cheese, molasses, yogurt, bone meal, dolomite, almonds, beef liver	Backache, bone loss, foot/leg cramps, heart palpitations, insomnia, muscle cramps, nervousness, obesity	Foetal requirements increase in last 3 months. Builds bones and teeth. Aids in muscle contraction, blood clotting, and regulation of heartbeat Regulates use of other minerals in the body.

Chromium	RDA: none stated SR: 100–300 mcg Toxicity: not known P&L: 50–200 mcg	Brewer's yeast, clams, corn oil, whole grain cereals	Atherosclerosis, glucose intolerance in diabetes, hypoglycemia	Aids in glucose regulation and carbohydrate metabolism.
Copper	RDA: 2 mg SR: 2–4 mg Toxicity: not known P&L: 2–4 mg	Legumes, nuts, organ meats, seafood, raisins, molasses, bone meal, Brazil nuts, soybeans	**Anaemia, impaired respiration, weakness**	Forms protective myelin sheath on nerves. Aids in energy metabolism. Augments zinc functions.
Fluoride	RDA: 1.5–4.0 mg SR: none stated Toxicity: none stated P&L: 1.5–4.0 mg	Apples, beef, eggs, fish, milk, sardines	Weak bones and teeth	Aids in strengthening bones and teeth. Adds to calcium utilization. Protects against magnesium deficiency
Iodine	RDA: 100–150 mcg SR: 100–1,000 mcg Toxicity: not known P&L: 175–200 mcg	Seafood, kelp tablets, salt (iodized)	Atherosclerosis, cold hands and feet, goitre, hyperthyroidism, nervousness, obesity	Controls rate of energy usage. Aids in production of thyroxin.
Iron	RDA: 10–18 mg SR: 15–50 mg Toxicity: 100 P&L: 30–60 mg	Blackstrap molasses, eggs, fish, organ meats, poultry, wheat germ, dessicated liver, shredded wheat	**Anaemia, breathing difficulties, colitis, pale skin, fatigue, constipation**	Foetal requirements increase tenfold during last 6 weeks of pregnancy. Combines with protein to form haemoglobin. Aids mother in sustaining energy levels.

Vitamin/Mineral	Daily Dosage	Sources	Deficiency Symptoms	Benefits
Magnesium	RDA: 300-350 mg SR: 300-350 mg Toxicity: 30,000 mg P&L: 450 mg	Bran, honey, green vegetables, nuts, seafood, spinach, bone meal, kelp tablets, bran flakes, peanuts (roasted with skin), tuna fish (canned)	Depression, disorientation, heart conditions, irritability, kidney stones, nervousness, neuromuscular disorders, sensitivity to noise, stomach acidity, obesity, tremors	Aids in calcium functions. Coenzyme in energy and protein metabolism. Helps cellular metabolism, muscle actions, and tissue growth.
Manganese	RDA: 300-350 mg SR: 300-350 mg Toxicity: none stated P&L: none stated	Bananas, bran, celery, cereals, egg yolks, green leafy vegetables, legumes, liver, nuts, pineapples, whole grains	Ataxia (muscle coordination failure), allergies, asthma, diabetes, fatigue	Aids in production of insulin and prevention of muscular disorders.
Molybdenum	RDA: 150-500 mcg SR: none stated Toxicity: none stated P&L: 150-500 mcg	Meats, grains, legumes, green leafy vegetables	None ever reported. Oversupplementation can cause copper deficiency.	Mobilizes iron from the liver. Aids in removal of nitrogenous waste through urea.
Phosphorus	RDA: 800-1,200 mg SR: 1,000-1,400 mg Toxicity: not known Average daily intake: 1,200-1,600 mg P&L: none stated	Eggs, fish, grains, organ meats, meat, poultry, yellow cheese, calf liver, milk/yogurt, eggs (cooked)	Appetite loss, fatigue, irregular breathing, nervous disorders, obesity, stunted growth in children, stress, tooth and gum disorders, weight loss	Helps build bones and teeth.

Potassium	RDA: none stated SR: 100–300 mg Toxicity: not known Average daily intake: 1,950–5,850 mg P&L: none stated	Dates, figs, peaches, tomato juice, blackstrap molasses, peanuts, raisins, seafood, apricots (dried), bananas, flounder (baked), potatoes (baked), sunflower seeds	Allergies, colic in infants, constipation, diabetes, high blood pressure, heart disease (angina pectoris, congestive heart failure, myocardial infarction), general weakness, insomnia, muscle damage, nervousness, irregular heartbeat	With sodium, responsible for proper muscle contraction.
Selenium	RDA: 50–200 mcg SR: none stated Toxicity: none stated P&L: 50–200 mcg	Fish, whole grains, organ meats, cereals, Brazil nuts	Heart disease, muscular aches and pains, rapid aging	Protects cells against oxidation. Aids heart function. Helps synthesize protein in both liver and red blood cells. May protect against cancer. May protect against cot death.
Sodium	RDA: none stated SR: 100–300 mg Toxicity: 14,000 mg Average daily intake: 2,800–6,900 P&L: not known	Salt, milk, cheese, seafood	Appetite loss, dehydration, fever, intestinal gas, muscle shrinkage, vomiting, weight loss	With potassium, responsible for proper muscle contraction.

Vitamin/Mineral	Daily Dosage	Sources	Deficiency Symptoms	Benefits
Sulphur	RDA: none stated SR: trace Toxicity: not known P&L: not known	Bran, cheese, clams, eggs, nuts, fish, wheat germ	Skin orders (eczema, dermatitis, psoriasis)	Aids in production of haemoglobin. Is a component of protein and assists in all its functions.
Zinc	RDA: 15 mg SR: 20–100 mg Toxicity: not known P&L: 20–25 mg	Brewer's yeast, liver, seafood, soyabeans, spinach, sunflower seeds, mushrooms	Atherosclerosis, cirrhosis, delayed sexual maturity, diabetes, fatigue, foetal skeletal and nervous system malfunctions, high cholesterol level, loss of taste, poor appetite, prolonged wound healing, retarded growth, sterility	Important component in growth of skeletal system and nervous system. Component of insulin.

RDA, Recommended Dietary Allowance; *IU*, International Units; *SR*, Supplemental Range; *Mg*, Milligrams; *P&L*, Pregnant & Lactating; *Mcg*, Micrograms.

Appendix B: Nutrient Interactions

Vitamin/Mineral	Protagonist	Antagonist
A	Vitamin B complex, Choline, Vitamin C, Vitamin D, Vitamin E, Unsaturated fatty acids, Calcium, Phosphorus, Zinc.	Air Pollution, Alcohol, Arsenicals, Aspirin, Corticosteroid drugs (eg. prednisone and cortisone), Dicoumarol, Mineral oil, Nitrates, Phenobarbital, Thyroid gland.
B Complex	Vitamin C, Vitamin E, Calcium, Phosphorus.	Alcohol, Antibiotics, Aspirin, Corticosteroid drugs, Diuretics.
B1 (Thiamine)	Vitamin B complex, Vitamin B2 (riboflavin), Folic acid, Niacin, Vitamin C, Vitamin E, Manganese, Sulphur.	Alcohol, Antibiotics, Excess sugar.
B2 (Riboflavin)	Vitamin B complex, Vitamin B6, Niacin, Vitamin C	Alcohol, Antibiotics, Oral contraceptives
Niacin (B3)	Vitamin B Complex Vitamin B1 (thiamine), Vitamin B2 (riboflavin) Vitamin C	Alcohol, Antibiotics, Excess sugar.
Pantothenic Acid (B5)	Vitamin B complex, Vitamin B6 (pyridoxine), Vitamin B12, Biotin, Folic acid, Vitamin C, Calcium, Sulphur	Aspirin, Methylbromide (an insecticide fumigant for some foods).
B5 (Pyridoxine)	Vitamin B complex, Vitamin B1 (thiamine), Vitamin B2 (riboflavin), Pantothenic acid, Vitamin C, Magnesium, Potassium, Linoleic acid, Sodium	Cortisone, Oestrogen, Oral contraceptives.

B12	Vitamin B complex, Vitamin B6 (pyridoxine), Choline, Folic acid, Inositol, Vitamin C, Calcium, Iron, Potassium, Sodium	Dilantin, Oral contraceptives.
Pangamic Acid (B15)	Vitamin B complex, Vitamin C, Vitamin E.	
Biotin	Vitamin B complex, Vitamin B12, Folic acid, Pantothenic acid, Vitamin C, Sulphur	Antibiotics, Avidin (from raw egg whites), Sulphur drugs.
Choline	Vitamin A, Vitamin B complex, Vitamin B12, Folic acid, Inositol, Linoleic acid	Alcohol, Excess sugar.
Folic Acid	Vitamin B complex, Vitamin B12, Biotin, Pantothenic acid, Vitamin C	Alcohol, Anticonvulsants, Oral contraceptives, Phenobarbital.
Inositol	Vitamin B complex, Vitamin B12, Choline, Vitamin C, Vitamin E, Linoleic acid	Antibiotics.
Para-Amino-benzoic Acid (PABA)	Vitamin B complex, Folic acid, Vitamin C	Sulphur drugs.
C	All vitamins and minerals, Bioflavonoids, Calcium, Magnesium	Alcohol, Antibiotics, Antihistamines, Aspirin, Baking soda, Barbiturates, Cortisone, DDT, Oestrogen, Oral contraceptives, Petroleum, Smoking, Sulfonamides.
D	Vitamin A, Choline, Vitamin C, Unsaturated fatty acids, Calcium, Phosphorus	Alcohol, Corticosteroid drugs, Oral contraceptives, Dilantin.
E	Vitamin A, Vitamin B complex, Vitamin B1 (thiamine), Inositol, Vitamin C, Unsaturated fatty acids, Manganese, Selenium	Air pollution, Antibiotics, Chlorine, Hypolipidemic drugs, (cholesterol-lowering drugs), Inorganic iron, Mineral oil, Oral

		contraceptives, Rancid fats and oils.
K		Air pollution, Antibiotics, Anticoagulants, Mineral oil, Radiation, Rancid oils and fats.
Bioflavonoids (Vitamin P)	Vitamin C.	
Calcium	Vitamin A, Vitamin C, Vitamin D, Unsaturated fatty acids, Iron, Magnesium, Manganese, Phosphorus, Hydrochloric acid	Aspirin, Corticosteroid drugs, Thyroid.
Copper	Cobalt, Iron, Zinc.	
Iron	Vitamin B12, Folic acid, Vitamin C, Calcium, Cobalt, Copper, Phosphorus, Hydrochloric acid	Antacids, Aspirin, EDTA (a food preservative), Vitamin E.
Magnesium	Vitamin B6, Vitamin C, Vitamin D, Calcium, Phosphorus, Protein	Alcohol, Corticosteroid drugs, Diuretics.
Manganese	Vitamin B1 (thiamine), Vitamin E, Calcium, Phosphorus	Antibiotics.
Phosphorus	Vitamin A, Vitamin D, Unsaturated fatty acids, Calcium, Iron, Manganese, Protein	Alcohol, Antacids, Aspirin, Corticosteriod drugs, Diuretics, Thyroid.
Potassium	Vitamin B6, Sodium	Aspirin, Corticosteroid drugs, Diuretics, Sodium.
Selenium	Vitamin E.	
Sodium	Vitamin D.	
Sulphur	Vitamin B complex, Vitamin B1 (thiamine), Biotin, Pantothenic acid.	

Zinc	Vitamin A, Vitamin B6, Vitamin E, Calcium, Copper, Phosphorus	Alcohol, Chelating compounds (used to remove excess copper), Corticosteriod drugs, Diuretics, Oral contraceptives.

There is no data for Chlorine, Chromium, Fluorine, Iodine or Molybdenum.

Appendix C: Recommendations for Exercise

- Always use correct posture, form, and technique, and always wear trainers or aerobic shoes to reduce the risk of foot, ankle, or leg injuries.
- Stand with the head level, back straight, abdomen tucked in, pelvis tilted forward, and knees slightly bent.
- Always warm up for 7-10 minutes before exercising strenuously. Be sure to use slow, rhythmic, large muscle group activities. This will increase the blood flow to the muscles and raise the core temperature. Also, cool down in a manner similar to the warm-up.
- Flexibility exercises should consist of only range-of-motion or static stretching. These should be performed during the last portion of the warm-up and cool-down periods. Never use bouncing motions or ballistic stretching to increase flexibility.
- Perform flexibility, calisthenic, and aerobic activities during each exercise session.
- Exhale on the exertion phase of the movement.
- Perform fewer repetitions per set and more sets of an exercise rather than going for the 'burn.'
- Never lock the knees for any stretching exercise.
- Always bend forward from the waist and go no farther than a flat-back position, to protect the lower back.
- Refrain from using momentum to complete an exercise or to change direction during an exercise. Perform all exercises slowly, so the muscles can receive the maximum benefit.
- Do not perform any activities that require unnatural twisting of the back, such as the standard windmill toe touch.
- During squats and lunges, keep the head level, back straight, buttocks higher than the knees, and the knees directly over the toes.
- During hip and side-leg work, rest on the hip and the forearm.
- During side bends, keep the opposite hip in, and the near shoulder over the ankle.
- The abdomen should be tucked in during all sit-up exercises.
- Never hyperextend the back or any joint.
- Stretch a muscle group after it has been worked.

- During aerobics and cool-down, always maintain an upright posture with the head above the heart.
- During jumping exercises, make sure you land on the toes, then the ball of the foot, and finally the heel, so the shock wave is spread throughout the foot. Never land only on the toes.
- Exercises should be performed at least three times a week, but there is no reason that some type of exercise cannot be performed every day.
- Previously sedentary individuals should begin an exercise program slowly and proceed at their own rate. This will minimize the chance of injuries, overexertion, and undue fatigue.
- Follow your own exercise prescription. Do not compete with or try to match the progress of others. Always stay within your target heart-rate zone.
- Never go immediately from a static position (sitting or reclining) to a high level of vigorous activity, or vice versa.
- Supplement your exercise program with regular walking at least three times a week, and preferably at a pace that elevates your heart rate into its training zone.
- Set reasonable health and fitness goals for yourself that require some effort but that you are capable of achieving. Do not expect instant results, because fitness benefits require about one or two months to become noticeable.

25 Exercises Not to Do

Exercise	Injury-prone areas
Hurdler stretch	Knee, lower back
Plough	Neck
Back arch (hyperextension)	Lower back
Neck hyperextensions	Atlas and axis vertebrae compression
Cobra	Lower back
Straight leg stretch	Hamstrings, lower back
Straight-leg sit-up	Lower back
Straight-leg side bend	Hips, lower back
Double leg raises	Lower back
Prone-back leg raises	Lower back
Side bends, both arms overhead	Hips, lower back

Rocking cradles (rockers)	Lower back
Deep lunges, deep squats	Knee
High donkey kicks with neck hyperextension	Lower back, knee, neck
Shoulder stand (bicycles)	Shoulders, neck
Full-range sit-up	Lower back
Low-leg scissors	Lower back
Double knee stretch (standing heel-to-butt stretch)	Knees
Back/neck hyperextension	Back, neck
Jumping jacks	Heels, ankles, knees
Jackknife sit-ups	Lower back
High pelvic tilts	Lower back, neck, shoulders
Swans	Hips, lower back
Hip rolls/hip swings	Hips, lower back
Windmill toe touches	Lower back, knees, hamstrings

Proper Sequencing of Exercise

Warm-Up: 7–10 Minutes

- Begin with low-intensity, rhythmic activities.
- Use range-of-motion activities.
- Use static stretching during the last phase of warm-up.

Conditioning/Calisthenics: 20–23 Minutes

- Proceed from standing posture to floor posture.
- Work muscle groups in sequence. Do not go back and forth from abdomen to legs to hips to abdomen, etc.
- Use static stretching during this phase, especially after a muscle group has been worked.
- Do not work for the 'burn.' Less repetitions per set and more sets will provide the necessary conditioning effect, as well as keep the workout more enjoyable because of less pain.
- Vary the calisthenic exercises to work all the muscle groups and prevent boredom.
- Do not use twisting, ballistic, or momentum-type movements.

Conditioning/Aerobics: 20–23 Minutes

- Begin with moderate intensity and build up as the period progresses. Work both the upper and lower body.
- Take pulse checks every 5-7 minutes.
- Know your own capabilities. Choose a class designed for your skill level.
- Never place the head below the heart.
- Never go down to the floor or bend all the way over.
- Never completely stop moving.
- Use music that is continuous, upbeat, recognizable, and enjoyable.

Cool-Down: 7–10 Minutes

- Use activities that are similar to the warm-up.
- Do not go down to the floor to stretch. Do standing stretches.
- Make a final pulse check and keep the ending pulse rate at or below 60 percent of the maximum heart rate.